NOURISH YOUR KIDNEYS: THE ESSENTIAL COOKBOOK FOR RENAL HEALTH

DELICIOUS AND NUTRITIOUS RECIPES FOR MANAGING KIDNEY DISEASE, IMPROVING DIET, AND ENHANCING OVERALL WELLBEING

———————

Zera Perry

ZERA PERRY

NOURISH YOUR KIDNEYS: THE ESSENTIAL COOKBOOK FOR RENAL HEALTH
Copyright © 2022 by Zera Perry

TABLE OF CONTENTS

AUTHOR BIO

Zera Perry, a culinary visionary and advocate for holistic well-being, brings a wealth of knowledge and passion to the world of nutrition. With a background deeply rooted in understanding the intricate dynamics of health, Zera has become a guiding force in promoting well-being through mindful eating.

Her culinary journey began as more than a pursuit of flavors; it was a mission to reshape the narrative surrounding food and its impact on health. Zera's dedication to fostering well-being is reflected not only in her insightful approach to understanding health conditions but also in her commitment to empowering individuals to make informed choices. Navigating the nuances of dietary intricacies, Zera skillfully emphasizes the importance of a balanced lifestyle without restrictive measures. Her approach showcases that one can enjoy delicious and healthful meals without compromising on taste.

Zera stands as a beacon of empowerment for individuals seeking to enhance their overall health. Her writing transcends the confines of a cookbook, serving as a celebration of positive lifestyle choices. Zera encourages readers to take charge of their health journey, providing valuable insights and tools to nourish both body and spirit.

Embark on a journey with Zera Perry, where each interaction is an opportunity to discover the joys of a holistic and health-conscious lifestyle. Let Zera's wisdom be your guide on the path to a healthier, happier you.

INTRODUCTION

Step into a world of culinary wellness with "Nourish Your Kidneys: The Essential Cookbook for Renal Health." This meticulously crafted cookbook extends a warm invitation to individuals navigating the intricacies of kidney disease or impaired kidney function. My mission is clear – to provide not just a cookbook, but a companion on your journey to optimal health. Tailored with precision to meet the unique dietary requirements of those with kidney-related conditions, this cookbook is your guide to supporting kidney health and elevating overall well-being through a symphony of flavorful and kidney-friendly recipes.

Embark on a journey that unravels the critical role your kidneys play in eliminating excess fluids and waste products from your body. As we delve into the core of "Nourish Your Kidneys," the narrative unfolds with a crucial understanding: when kidney function is compromised, dietary adjustments become the cornerstone of maintaining resilience and achieving optimal health. The cookbook stresses the significance of restricting Sodium, Potassium, and Phosphorus, while highlighting the pivotal role of quality protein in crafting a well-balanced diet.

Turn the pages of this cookbook, and you'll be greeted by a myriad of healthy and delectable recipes meticulously aligned with the requirements of a renal diet. Each recipe is an artful creation, promising not just nourishment but a delightful symphony of flavors and textures. Precision is our mantra – every recipe is designed with a keen eye on maintaining low levels of Sodium, Potassium, and Phosphorus. Detailed nutritional breakdowns, portion sizes, and crystal-clear instructions beckon you into the realm of appetizers, main courses, side dishes, and desserts. Feel the empowerment to experiment with new flavors, cook meals that not only tantalize your taste buds but also nurture your kidneys, and revel in the joy of the culinary process.

Whether you stand at the threshold of a recent kidney disease diagnosis or aspire to refine your dietary choices for enhanced kidney function, "Nourish Your Kidneys" stands as a beacon of knowledge and flavor. It isn't just a cookbook; it's a catalyst for a positive and enjoyable approach to managing a renal diet. Empowering individuals with kidney-related conditions, it encourages you to seize control of your health through the delectable gateway of kidney-friendly recipes. Welcome to a culinary adventure where nourishing your kidneys is not just a journey but a celebration of health and flavor!

CHAPTER 1: BREAKFAST AND BRUNCH

Welcome to the opening chapter, where we explore the world of Breakfast and Brunch. In this section, you'll discover a delectable array of kidney-friendly recipes meticulously crafted to support your renal health journey. From the inviting scent of Kidney-Friendly Pumpkin Waffles to the savory satisfaction of a Herb-infused Omelet, each dish represents a tasteful stride towards nurturing your kidneys while ensuring a delightful culinary experience. This compilation goes beyond mere recipes; it signifies a dedication to prioritizing your well-being right from the beginning of your day. Whether you choose the comforting warmth of Walnut Porridge, the invigorating sip of a Berry Cleanser Smoothie, or the wholesome goodness of Low-Phosphorus Whole-Grain Pancakes, each offering plays a role in maintaining the crucial balance essential for renal health. Embark on this flavorful journey through breakfast and brunch, embracing a symphony of tastes that align with your commitment to kidney health.

KIDNEY-FRIENDLY PUMPKIN WAFFLES

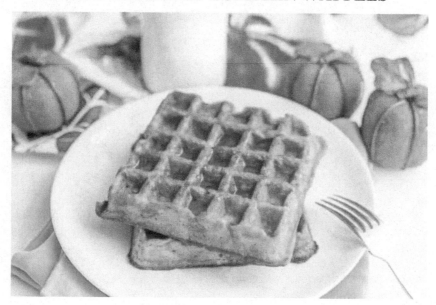

Makes: 4

INGREDIENTS:

☐ ½ cup almond flour

☐ ½ cup coconut flour

☐ 1 teaspoon baking powder

☐ 1½ teaspoons ground cinnamon

☐ ¾ teaspoon ground ginger

☐ ½ teaspoon ground cloves

☐ ½ teaspoon ground nutmeg

☐ 2 tablespoons olive oil

☐ 5 organic eggs

☐ ¾ cup almond milk

☐ ½ cup pumpkin purée

☐ 2 bananas, peeled and sliced

☐ Pinch Low-Sodium Salt

INSTRUCTIONS:

a) Start by preheating the waffle maker and greasing it lightly.

b) Blend all the ingredients together in a blender until they are thoroughly combined.

c) Transfer the mixture to the waffle maker and let it cook for around 5 minutes.

NUTRITION PER SERVING:

Calories: 369 | Fat: 22.5g | Carbohydrates: 31g | Fiber: 10.8g | Sugars: 8.8 g | Protein: 14.1g | Sodium 120 mg | Potassium: 150-250mg | Phosphorus: 100-150mg

HERB-INFUSED OMELET

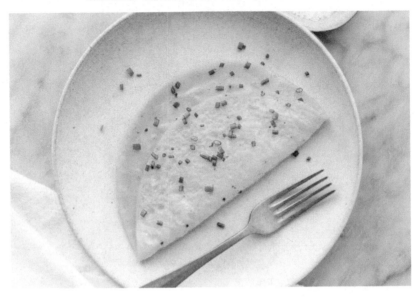

Makes: 2 Servings

INGREDIENTS:

☐4 large eggs

☐¼ cup low-Phosphorus milk substitute (such as almond milk)

☐¼ teaspoon salt substitute (such as Potassium chloride)

☐¼ teaspoon dried herbs of your choice (e.g., thyme, oregano, or basil)

☐¼ teaspoon black pepper

☐1 teaspoon olive oil

INSTRUCTIONS:

a)Crack the eggs into a bowl, add the low-phosphorus milk substitute, and whisk well.

b)Stir in the salt substitute, dried herbs, and black pepper.

c)Heat the olive oil in a non-stick skillet over medium heat. Pour the egg mixture into the skillet, allowing it to spread evenly. Cook the omelet for 2-3 minutes or until the edges start to set.

d)Using a spatula, gently lift the edges of the omelet, allowing any uncooked egg to flow underneath.

e)Continue cooking until the omelet is mostly set but still slightly runny on top. Carefully fold the omelet in half using the spatula. Cook for an additional 1-2 minutes until the omelet is fully set but still moist.

f)Slide the herb-infused omelet onto a plate and serve immediately.

NUTRITION PER SERVING:

Calories: 25 Calories: | Protein: 2 grams | Fat: 1.5 grams | Carbohydrates: Less than 1 gram | Phosphorus: 20mg | Sodium: 20mg | Potassium: 40 milligrams

WALNUT PORRIDGE

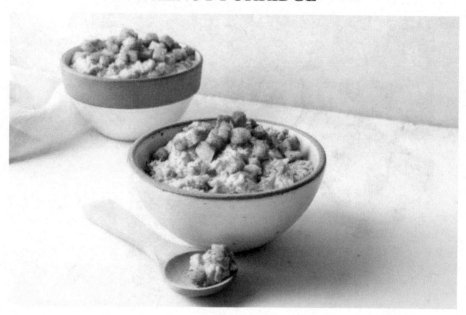

Makes: 5

INGREDIENTS:

☐½ cup pecans

☐½ cup almonds

☐¼ cup sunflower seeds

☐¼ cup chia seeds

☐¼ cup unsweetened coconut flakes

☐4 cups unsweetened almond milk

☐½ teaspoon cinnamon powder

☐¼ teaspoon ginger powder

☐1 teaspoon powdered stevia

☐1 tablespoon almond butter

INSTRUCTIONS:

a)Finely blend pecans, almonds, and sunflower seeds.

b)In a skillet, combine the blended nut mix, chia seeds, coconut flakes, almond milk, spices, and stevia, then bring the mixture to a gentle boil. Let it simmer for 20 minutes.

c)When serving, accompany the dish with a spoonful of almond butter.

NUTRITION PER SERVING:

Calories: 292 | Fat: 7.5g | Carbohydrates: 9.6g | Fiber: 6.5g | Sugars: 1.2g | Protein: 8g | Sodium 121 mg | Phosphorus: 150-200mg | Potassium: 200-300mg

BERRY CLEANSER SMOOTHIE

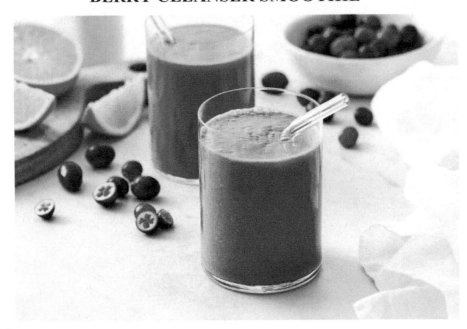

Makes: 2 Servings

INGREDIENTS:

☐3 Swiss chard leaves, stems removed

☐¼ cup frozen cranberries

☐1 cup of raspberries

☐2 pitted Medjool date

☐2 tablespoons ground flaxseed

☐1 cup of water

INSTRUCTIONS:

a)Combine all the ingredients and blend until a smooth consistency is achieved.

NUTRITION PER SERVING:

Calories: 202.4 | Fat 4.5 g | Saturated Fat 2 g | Cholesterol 0.0 mg | Sodium 37 mg | Protein 13g | Carbohydrate 33 g | Dietary Fiber 9.6 g | Sugars 11 g | Phosphorus: 50-100mg | Potassium: 300-400mg

LOW-PHOSPHORUS WHOLE-GRAIN PANCAKES

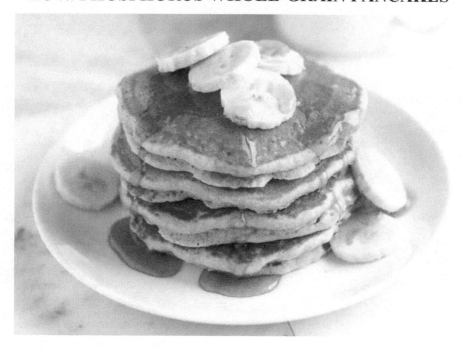

Makes: 2

INGREDIENTS:

☐ 1 cup whole wheat flour

☐ 1 tablespoon sugar or a sugar substitute

☐ 1 teaspoon baking powder (look for a brand with low Sodium content)

☐ ½ teaspoon baking soda

☐ ¼ teaspoon salt substitute (such as Potassium chloride)

☐ 1 cup low-Phosphorus milk substitute (such as almond milk)

☐ 1 large egg

☐ 1 tablespoon oil (such as olive oil or canola oil)

INSTRUCTIONS:

a)Combine whole wheat flour, sugar (or substitute), baking powder, baking soda, and salt substitute.

b)Whisk low-Phosphorus milk substitute, egg, and oil in a separate bowl.

c)Pour wet ingredients into dry, and stir until just mixed. Allow batter to rest for 5 minutes.

d)Pour ¼ cup batter onto a greased skillet. Cook until bubbles appear, then flip and cook until golden brown (1-2 minutes). Use the remaining batter, adding oil if needed.

e)Enjoy warm, kidney-friendly, low-Phosphorus, low-Sodium pancakes with kidney-friendly toppings.

NUTRITION PER SERVING:

Calories: 100 | Carbohydrates: 12 grams | Protein: 4 grams | Fat: 2.4 grams | Fiber: 2 grams | Potassium: 100 mg | Sodium: 80 mg | Phosphorus: 50 mg

LOW-PHOSPHOROUS OATMEAL

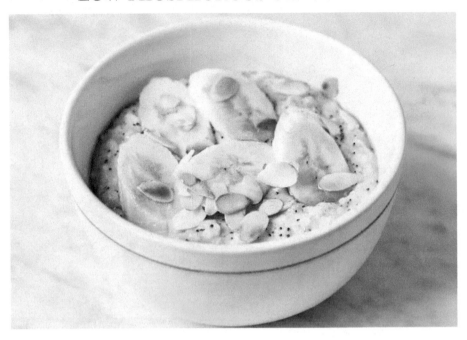

Makes: 2

INGREDIENTS:

☐½ cup old-fashioned oats

☐1 cup water

☐½ cup low-fat milk (or milk substitute)

☐1 tablespoon honey or sweetener of your choice (optional)

☐¼ teaspoon cinnamon (optional)

☐Toppings of your choice (e.g., fresh fruits, nuts, seeds)

INSTRUCTIONS:

a)Combine the oats and water in a saucepan.

b)Heat the mixture over medium heat until it reaches a boiling point.

c)Reduce the heat to low and let it simmer for 5 minutes, stirring occasionally.

d)Add the low-fat milk, honey (or sweetener), and cinnamon (if preferred) to the saucepan.

e)Continue cooking for an additional 2-3 minutes, or until the oatmeal reaches the desired consistency, stirring occasionally. Take the saucepan off the heat and allow it to cool for a few minutes.

f)Transfer the oatmeal to a serving bowl and garnish it with your preferred toppings, such as fresh fruits, nuts, or seeds. Gently stir to combine everything and enjoy the warm oatmeal.

NUTRITION PER SERVING:

Calories: 150-200 | Carbohydrates: 25-30 grams | Protein: 6-8 grams | Fat: 2-4 grams | Fiber: 4-6 grams | Potassium: 150-200 mg | Sodium: 50-100 mg | Phosphorus: Less than 100 mg

NUT AND SEED GRANOLA

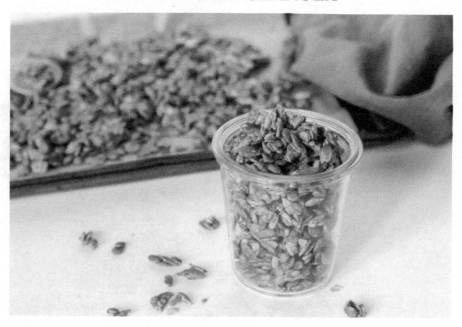

Makes: 2

INGREDIENTS:

☐ ¼ cup sunflower seeds, shelled

☐ 1 cup cashews

☐ pinch low Sodium salt

☐ ¼ cup pumpkin seeds, shelled

☐ ¾ cup almonds

☐ ½ cup unsweetened coconut flakes

☐ a few drops of stevia

☐ 1 teaspoon vanilla

INSTRUCTIONS:

a) Heat your oven to a temperature of 300 °F and arrange a baking sheet by placing a lining on it.

b) Pulse the cashews, almonds, coconut flakes, and pumpkin seeds.

c) Combine vanilla and stevia.

d) Combine the blended mixture and the sunflower seeds, stirring to guarantee that they are thoroughly coated. Evenly distribute the mixture onto the prepared baking sheet and bake for 25 minutes.

e) Remove it from the oven. Sprinkle salt onto the mixture.

f) Once it has adequately cooled, proceed to break it into individual pieces.

NUTRITION PER SERVING:

Calories: 260 | Protein 4.4 grams | Fat 2.9 grams | Carbohydrates 40.5 grams | Sodium 77 mg | Potassium: 200-300mg | Phosphorus: 150-250mg

APPLE CHIA DELIGHT

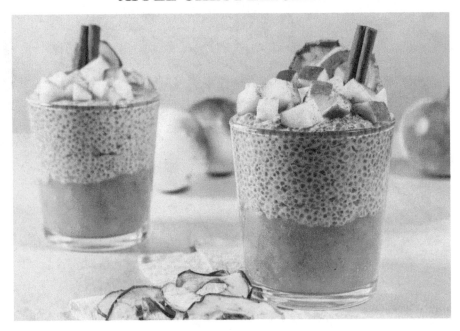

Makes: 2

INGREDIENTS:

☐½ chopped dried organic apple

☐2 cups organic chia seeds

☐1 cup organic hemp hearts

☐2 tablespoons real cinnamon

☐1 cup chopped nuts

☐1 teaspoon low Sodium salt

INSTRUCTIONS:

a)Combine all the ingredients, thoroughly mixing them together.

b)When serving, include a modest quantity of stevia as a final touch.

NUTRITION PER SERVING:

Calories: 150-200 | Fat: 4 grams | Saturated Fat: 0-1 gram | Sodium: 4mg | Potassium: 150-200mg | Carbohydrates: 25 grams | Sugars: 15-20 grams | Protein: 3-5 grams | Phosphorus: 80-120mg

PORRIDGE WITH CARAMELIZED BANANA AND PECANS

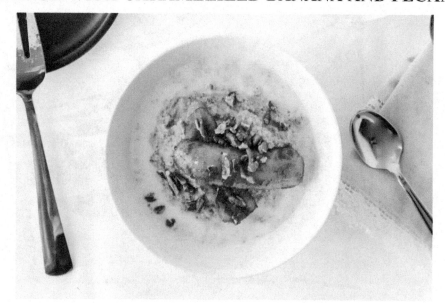

Makes: 2

INGREDIENTS:

☐1 cup raw pecans, soaked for 8 hours or overnight

☐1 cup raw cashews, soaked for 8 hours or overnight

☐2 cups unsweetened almond milk (low-phosphorus milk substitute)

☐4 Medjool dates, pitted

☐1 tablespoon chia seeds

☐1 teaspoon alcohol-free vanilla extract

☐¼ teaspoon sea salt (low-sodium option)

☐2 bananas, peeled, sliced in half, and lengthwise

☐1 tablespoon unsalted butter or ghee

☐1 ½ tablespoons sugar-free maple syrup

INSTRUCTIONS:

a)In a food processor, blend soaked nuts, dates, chia seeds, vanilla extract, and sea salt until finely ground.

b)Transfer nut mixture to a pot, add almond milk, heat until smooth, then remove from heat.

c)In a skillet, combine butter and sugar-free maple syrup, and cook bananas for 1 minute on each side.

d)Divide porridge into four bowls, and top with caramelized bananas. Serve immediately.

NUTRITION PER SERVING:

Calories: Per Serving: 290 | Fat 19g | Cholesterol 0mg | Sodium 10mg | Carbohydrates 28g | Sugars 18g | Protein 6g | Potassium: 400-500mg | Phosphorus: 200-250mg

QUINOA PORRIDGE

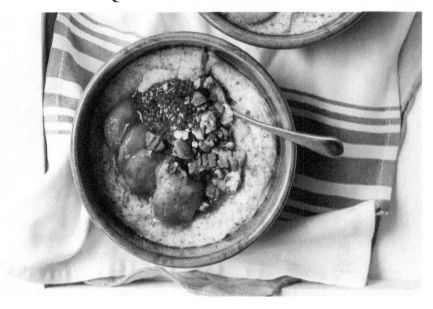

Makes: 4

INGREDIENTS:

☐2 cups of water

☐½ teaspoon organic vanilla extract

☐½ cup coconut milk

☐1 cup uncooked red quinoa, rinsed and drained

☐¼ teaspoon fresh lemon zest, finely grated

☐10-12 drops of liquid stevia

☐1 teaspoon ground cinnamon

☐½ teaspoon each ground ginger and ground nutmeg

☐Pinch of ground cloves

☐2 tablespoons almonds, chopped

INSTRUCTIONS:

a)Combine quinoa, water, and vanilla extract in a skillet and bring the mixture to a boil.

b)Lower the heat to a simmer and let it cook for approximately 15 minutes.

c)Stir in the coconut milk, lemon zest, stevia, and spices to the skillet with the quinoa.

d)Take the skillet off the heat and immediately fluff the quinoa using a fork.

e)Divide the quinoa mixture equally among serving bowls. Sprinkle with a garnish of chopped almonds.

NUTRITION PER SERVING:

Calories: 248 | Fat: 11.4g | Carbohydrates: 30.5g | Fiber: 4.4g | Sugars: 1.3g | Protein: 7.4g | Sodium 34.5 mg | Phosphorus: 150-200mg | Potassium: 150-200mg

KIDNEY-FRIENDLY CREPES

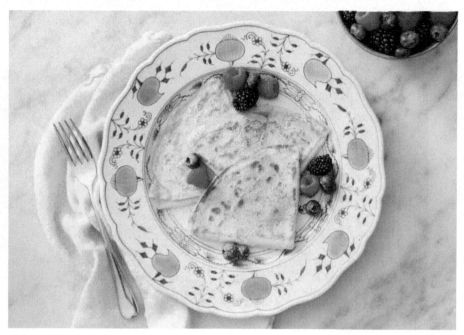

Makes: 2 Servings

INGREDIENTS:

☐1 cup all-purpose flour

☐1 cup low-Phosphorus milk (e.g., almond milk or rice milk)

☐2 large eggs

☐1 tablespoon kidney-friendly sweetener (e.g., erythritol or stevia)

☐½ teaspoon vanilla extract

☐Cooking spray or a small amount of butter for greasing the pan

INSTRUCTIONS:

a)Whisk together flour, low-Phosphorus milk, eggs, kidney-friendly sweetener, and vanilla extract until smooth. Rest the batter for 15 minutes.

b)Preheat a non-stick crepe pan over medium heat with cooking spray or a small amount of butter.

c)Pour ¼ cup batter into the pan, and swirl for even distribution.

d)Cook for 1-2 minutes until golden; flip and cook the other side.

e)Repeat with remaining batter, stacking cooked crepes.

f)Serve warm with kidney-friendly fillings like fresh berries, sliced bananas, or a sprinkle of cinnamon.

NUTRITION PER SERVING:

Calories: 80-100; Protein: 4-6 grams | Carbohydrates: 12-15 grams | Fat: 2-4 grams | Sodium: 50-70mg | Potassium: 60-80mg | Phosphorus: 80-100mg

PECAN PORRIDGE WITH BANANA

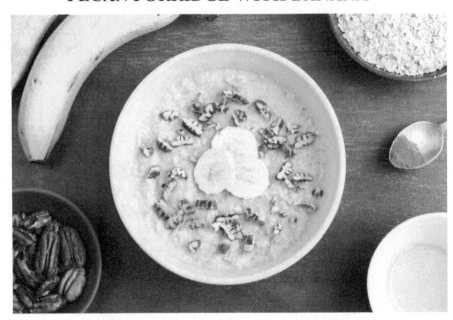

Makes: 2 Servings

INGREDIENTS:

☐ ½ cup soaked pecans

☐ ¾ cup boiling water

☐ ½ very ripe banana

☐ a few drops of a few drops of stevia

☐ 2 tablespoons coconut butter

☐ ½ teaspoon cinnamon

☐ ⅛ teaspoon sea salt

INSTRUCTIONS:

a) Blitz all the ingredients until they reach a texture of smoothness and creaminess.

b) Transfer the blended mixture to a pan and cook it over medium heat for approximately 5 minutes.
Serve and enjoy.

NUTRITION PER SERVING:

Calories: Per Serving: 290 | Total Fat 19g | Cholesterol 0mg | Sodium: 200-300mg | Total Carbohydrates 28g | Sugars 18g | Protein 6g | Phosphorus: 250-350mg | Potassium: 400-500mg

SPICY SWEET POTATO BREAKFAST BOWL

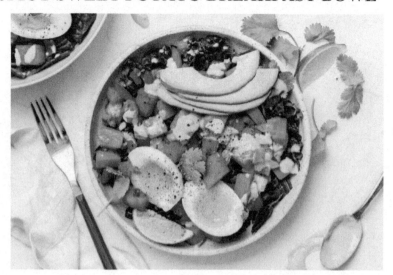

Makes: 4 Servings

INGREDIENTS:
FOR THE SWEET POTATO:
☐2 tablespoons avocado oil or extra virgin olive oil

☐2 medium sweet potatoes, chopped

☐½ sweet onion, chopped

☐1 red bell pepper, chopped

☐2 garlic cloves, minced

☐Low sodium salt and Pepper

OTHER INGREDIENTS
☐Kale, chopped and massaged (or spinach or mixed greens)

☐Avocado, sliced or chopped into small pieces

☐Hard-Boiled Eggs

☐Tahini Sauce (low-sodium) and Fresh Cilantro, chopped

INSTRUCTIONS:
a) Heat oil in a skillet. Add sweet potatoes and onions, and sprinkle with salt and pepper.

b) Stir to coat. Cover, lower heat, and cook for 15-20 minutes, stirring occasionally, until sweet potatoes are almost tender. Increase heat, and stir in bell pepper and garlic. Cook on high for 2-5 minutes until sweet potatoes are cooked through. Serve over kale, topped with avocado, eggs, and low-sodium tahini sauce.

c) Garnish with chopped cilantro.

NUTRITION PER SERVING:
Calories: 460 | Fat 23g grams | Saturated Fat 9g grams | Carbohydrates 24g grams | Fiber 4g grams | Sugars 7g grams | Protein 40g grams | Phosphorus: 250-350mg | Sodium: 300-400mg | Potassium: 600-800mg

BLUEBERRY CINNAMON BREAKFAST BAKE

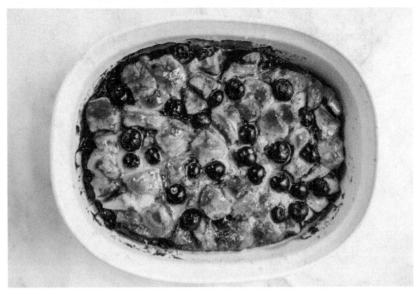

Makes: 6 Servings

INGREDIENTS:

☐2 teaspoons cinnamon, divided

☐2 eggs, beaten

☐¼ cup brown sugar, divided

☐8 slices of whole-wheat bread

☐1 cup of low-fat milk

☐3 cups blueberries

☐Zest of 1 lemon, divided

INSTRUCTIONS:

a)Preheat the oven to 350 °F (180 °C).

b)In a bowl, combine cinnamon, eggs, milk, brown sugar, and zest.

c)In another mixing bowl, toss the bread and blueberries with the egg mixture, whisking until the liquid is mostly absorbed. Transfer the batter into muffin tins. Sprinkle 1 tablespoon of brown sugar and 1 teaspoon of cinnamon over the French toast cups. Bake for approximately 18 minutes, or until the French toast is cooked and the top is nicely browned. Meanwhile, in a small saucepan, mix the remaining 1 cup of blueberries, lemon zest, and 1 tablespoon of brown sugar, and cook for about 10 minutes to release the juices. Gently crush the blueberries and spoon the syrupy blueberry mixture over the toasted French toast.

NUTRITION PER SERVING:

Calories: 170 | 3g Fat | 171mg Sodium | 30g Carbohydrates (4g fiber, 15g Sugar, 7g Added) | 7g Protein | Phosphorus: 200-300mg | Potassium: 200-300mg

GREEN TWIST SMOOTHIE

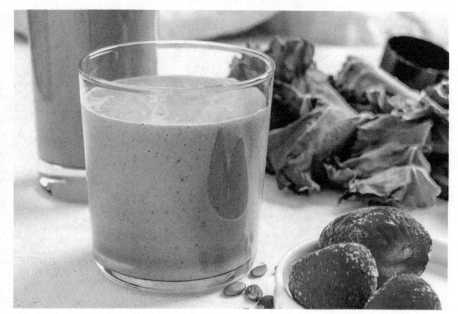

Makes: 2 Servings

INGREDIENTS:
☐1 cup kale, stems removed
☐1 cup dandelion greens
☐1 orange, peeled, seeds removed
☐2 cups strawberries
☐2 kiwis, peeled and chopped
☐½ tablespoon lemon juice
☐½ cup water

INSTRUCTIONS:
a)Place all the ingredients, excluding the purified water, into a blender.
b)Gradually add the purified water and ice to reach your desired consistency.
c)Blend until smooth.

NUTRITION PER SERVING:
Calories: 70 | Total Fat 0.5g | Carbohydrates 15g | Protein 1g | Sodium 39.2mg | Phosphorus: 50-100mg | Potassium: 300-400mg

BERRY PEACH SMOOTHIE

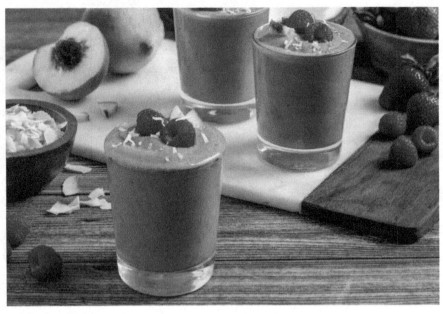

Makes: 2 servings

INGREDIENTS:

☐1 cup frozen mixed berries (blueberries, strawberries, raspberries)

☐1 ripe peach, peeled and sliced

☐½ cup low-fat Greek yogurt

☐1 tablespoon chia seeds

☐1 tablespoon honey (optional, adjust to taste)

☐1 cup water or almond milk

☐Ice cubes (optional)

INSTRUCTIONS:

a)In a blender, combine the frozen mixed berries, sliced peach, Greek yogurt, chia seeds, and honey.

b)Add water or almond milk to the blender.

c)Blend until smooth and creamy. If a thicker consistency is desired, add ice cubes and blend again.

d)Taste the smoothie and adjust the sweetness by adding more honey if necessary.

e)Pour the smoothie into glasses and serve immediately.

NUTRITION PER SERVING:

Calories: 150 | Protein: 7g | Fat: 3g | Carbohydrates: 28g | Fiber: 6g | Sodium: 30mg | Potassium: 280mg | Phosphorous: 120mg

VEGETABLE FRITTATA

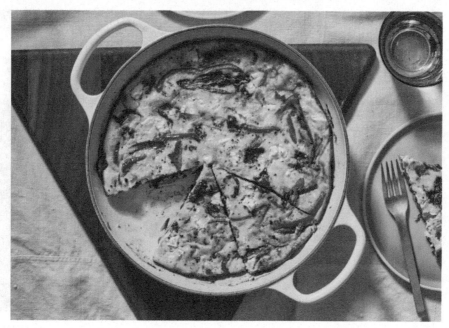

Makes: 4 servings

INGREDIENTS:

☐8 large eggs

☐¼ cup low-fat milk

☐1 cup diced zucchini

☐1 cup diced bell peppers (any color)

☐1 cup cherry tomatoes, halved

☐½ cup chopped spinach

☐¼ cup grated Parmesan cheese

☐Salt and pepper to taste

☐1 tablespoon olive oil

INSTRUCTIONS:

a)Preheat the oven to 350°F (180°C).

b)In a bowl, whisk together eggs, milk, Parmesan cheese, salt, and pepper. Heat olive oil in an oven-safe skillet over medium heat. Add zucchini, bell peppers, and spinach to the skillet. Sauté until vegetables are tender. Pour the egg mixture over the sautéed vegetables in the skillet. Arrange cherry tomatoes on top.

c)Cook on the stovetop for 2-3 minutes until the edges set. Transfer the skillet to the preheated oven and bake for 12-15 minutes or until the frittata is set in the center. Remove from the oven and cool before slicing.

NUTRITION PER SERVING:

Calories: 180 | Protein: 12g | Fat: 12g | Carbohydrates: 6g | Fiber: 2g | Sodium: 250mg | Potassium: 300mg | Phosphorous: 180mg

QUINOA BREAKFAST BOWL

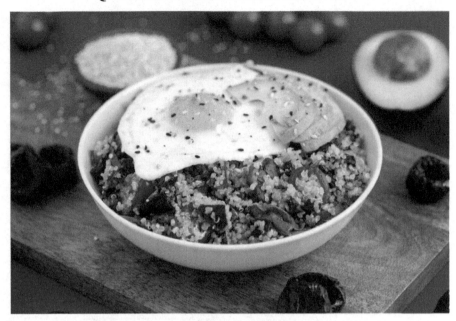

Makes: 2 bowls

INGREDIENTS:

☐ 1 cup quinoa
☐ 2 cups low-sodium vegetable broth
☐ 2 cups sliced baby bella or white button mushrooms (approx. 4 ounces), sliced
☐ 2 cups spinach, chopped
☐ 1 cup grape tomatoes, halved (approx. 5 ounces)
☐ 1 tablespoon olive oil
☐ ¼ teaspoon salt
☐ ¼ teaspoon black pepper
☐ 2 large eggs
☐ 1 large avocado, peeled and sliced

INSTRUCTIONS:

a)Rinse quinoa, and add to a pot with low-sodium vegetable broth. Bring to a boil, then simmer covered for 15 mins. Let sit covered for an additional 10 mins. Heat olive oil in a pan, sauté prepped vegetables with salt and pepper until cooked (about 10 mins). Set aside vegetables. In the same pan, fry eggs to your liking.

d)Slice avocado, and season with salt and pepper.

e)Assemble with layers of quinoa, sautéed vegetables, and egg. Top with avocado. Season to taste.

NUTRITION PER SERVING:

Calories: 450 | Protein: 16g | Fat: 24g | Carbohydrates: 45g | Fiber: 12g | Sodium: 300mg | Potassium: 850mg | Phosphorous: 200mg

SPINACH AND FETA BREAKFAST WRAP

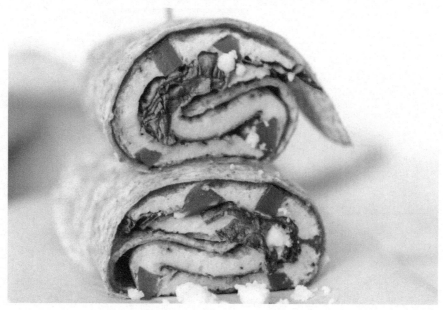

Makes: 1 serving

INGREDIENTS:

☐1 whole-grain tortilla

☐2 large eggs

☐¼ cup red pepper diced

☐1 handful of baby spinach

☐1 tablespoon goat feta cheese, crumbled

☐pinch of salt and pepper

INSTRUCTIONS:

a)Heat a medium frying pan on medium-high heat. Spray with olive oil.

b)In a medium bowl, whisk the eggs and add the peppers.

c)Pour the eggs and peppers into the skillet and season with salt and pepper. Cover and cook for 2 ½ minutes.

d)Remove the lid and top with spinach and feta. Fold in a half-moon shape, cover, and cook for 1 minute.

e)Transfer the omelet on top of the tortilla and wrap it up, burrito style.

f)Spray the pan with more oil, add the wrap, cook for 30 seconds, flip, and cook for another 30 seconds. Serve while warm.

NUTRITION PER SERVING:

Calories: 280 | Protein: 18g | Fat: 15g | Carbohydrates: 20g | Fiber: 3g | Sodium: 400mg | Potassium: 300mg | Phosphorous: 220mg

AVOCADO TOAST WITH TOMATO SALSA

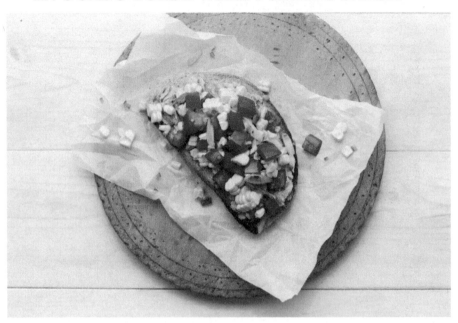

Makes: 1 serving

INGREDIENTS:

☐1 slice of whole-grain bread

☐½ avocado, mashed

☐1 small tomato, diced

☐1 tablespoon chopped cilantro

☐1 teaspoon lime juice

☐Salt and pepper to taste

INSTRUCTIONS:

a)Toast the bread slice.

b)Spread mashed avocado over the toast.

c)In a bowl, mix diced tomatoes, cilantro, lime juice, salt, and pepper to make salsa.

d)Top the avocado toast with tomato salsa.

NUTRITION PER SERVING:

Calories: 230 | Protein: 5g | Fat: 15g | Carbohydrates: 20g | Fiber: 8g | Sodium: 180mg | Potassium: 350mg | Phosphorous: 160mg

CHAPTER 2: APPETIZERS AND SNACKS

Welcome to Chapter 2, where we explore the world of Appetizers and Snacks. This chapter is a treasure trove of inventive and kidney-friendly delights, perfect for satisfying cravings between meals or impressing guests with healthy alternatives. From the savory punch of Low-Phosphorous Hummus to the crunchy goodness of Baked Sweet Potato Chips, these recipes are crafted to cater to your renal health needs without compromising on taste. Indulge in the vibrant flavors of Veggie and Sprout Rice Paper Rolls or the zesty kick of Jalapeño Popper Balls. Discover the wholesome goodness of Renal-Friendly Trail Mix and the satisfying crunch of Roasted Chickpeas Snack. Each recipe in this chapter is a testament to the belief that appetizers and snacks can be both delicious and supportive of your kidney health journey. So, whether you're craving the sweet notes of Date and Pistachio Bites, the savory elegance of Mini Portobello Pizzas, or the refreshing taste of Cucumber and Smoked Salmon Bites, these recipes invite you to savor the joy of snacking while prioritizing your renal well-being. Let's embark on this flavorful adventure through appetizers and snacks, where every bite contributes to the harmony of taste and health.

LOW-PHOSPHOROUS HUMMUS

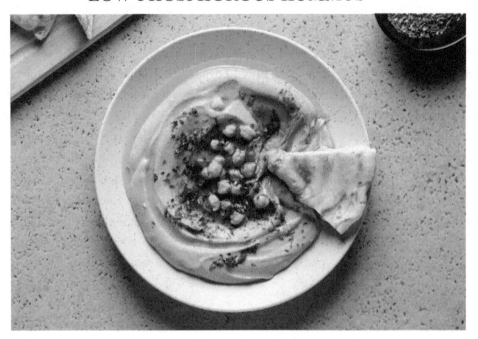

Makes: 6 Servings

INGREDIENTS:

☐1 can (15 ounces) low-Sodium chickpeas (garbanzo beans), drained and rinsed

☐2 tablespoons tahini (sesame seed paste)

☐2 tablespoons lemon juice

☐2 cloves garlic, minced

☐2 tablespoons olive oil

☐¼ teaspoon cumin (optional)

☐Salt and pepper to taste

☐Water (as needed to adjust consistency)

INSTRUCTIONS:

a)Combine chickpeas, tahini, lemon juice, garlic, olive oil, cumin (optional), salt, and pepper in a food processor or blender. Process the mixture until it becomes a smooth and creamy consistency.

b)Transfer the prepared hummus to a serving bowl.

c)For an optional garnish, drizzle a small amount of olive oil over the top and sprinkle with a pinch of cumin or paprika. Serve the homemade hummus alongside fresh vegetables, whole-grain crackers, or pita bread. Enjoy!

NUTRITION PER SERVING:

Calories: 60-80; Carbohydrates: 6-8 grams | Protein: 2-3 grams | Fat: 4-6 grams | Fiber: 1-2 grams | Potassium: 50-100 mg | Sodium: 50-100 mg | Phosphorus: Less than 50 mg

KIDNEY-FRIENDLY VEGETABLE DIP

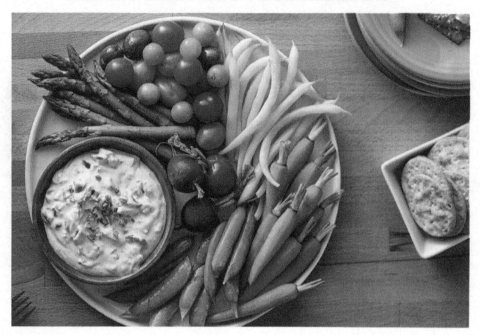

Makes: 2 Servings

INGREDIENTS:

☐1 cup low-fat sour cream or Greek yogurt

☐2 tablespoons chopped fresh dill (or 2 teaspoons dried dill)

☐1 tablespoon lemon juice

☐¼ teaspoon garlic powder

☐¼ teaspoon onion powder

☐¼ teaspoon salt

☐Freshly ground black pepper to taste

☐Assorted kidney-friendly vegetables for dipping (e.g., cucumber slices, bell pepper strips, carrot sticks, celery sticks, cherry tomatoes)

INSTRUCTIONS:

a)In a mixing bowl, combine low-fat sour cream or Greek yogurt, freshly chopped dill (or dried dill), lemon juice, garlic powder, onion powder, salt, and black pepper.

b)Seal the bowl with plastic wrap and refrigerate it for a minimum of 1 hour.

c)Arrange the assortment of kidney-friendly vegetables around the dip bowl on a platter or plate.

d)Present the dip alongside the vegetables for a delectable and kidney-friendly snack or appetizer.

NUTRITION PER SERVING:

Calories: 30-50; Carbohydrates: 2-4 grams | Protein: 2-4 grams | Fat: 1-2 grams | Fiber: 0 grams | Potassium: 50-100 mg | Sodium: 70-100 mg | Phosphorus: Less than 50 mg

BAKED SWEET POTATO CHIPS

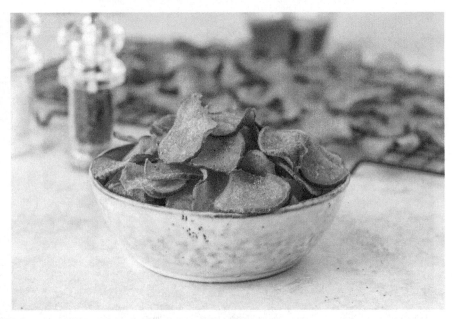

Makes: 2 Servings

INGREDIENTS:

☐2 medium sweet potatoes

☐1 tablespoon olive oil

☐Salt substitute (optional)

☐Herbs and spices of your choice (e.g., paprika, garlic powder, onion powder)

INSTRUCTIONS:

a)Preheat oven to 375°F (190°C), and prepare a baking sheet with parchment paper.

b)Wash and dry sweet potatoes.

c)Use a mandoline slicer to cut thin, uniform slices (⅛-inch thickness).

d)Toss slices in a bowl with olive oil for a light coating.

e)Optionally, sprinkle with salt substitute or preferred low-sodium herbs/spices.

f)Arrange slices on the baking sheet in a single layer.

g)Bake for 15-20 mins until edges turn golden and chips are crispy.

h)Remove from oven, let chips cool on the sheet to crisp up.

i)Transfer cooled chips to a serving bowl or storage container.

j)Repeat with remaining slices.

NUTRITION PER SERVING:

Calories: 100-120; Carbohydrates: 20-25 grams | Protein: 1-2 grams | Fat: 2-3 grams | Fiber: 3-4 grams | Potassium: 300-350 mg | Sodium: Less than 50 mg | Phosphorus: Less than 50 mg

CRISPY KALE CHIPS

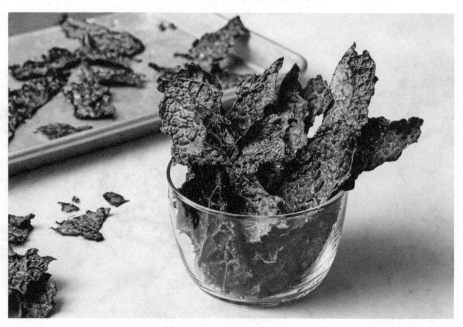

Makes: 2 servings

INGREDIENTS:
☐2 cups kale, washed and torn into bite-sized pieces
☐½ tablespoon olive oil
☐¼ teaspoon garlic powder
☐Salt and pepper to taste

INSTRUCTIONS:
a)Preheat the oven to 350°F (175°C).
b)In a bowl, toss kale with olive oil, garlic powder, salt, and pepper until well-coated.
c)Spread the kale in a single layer on a baking sheet.
d)Bake for 10-15 minutes or until the edges are crisp but not burnt.
e)Allow to cool and enjoy these flavorful and nutritious vegetable-based snacks.

NUTRITION PER SERVING:
Calories: 50| Protein: 2g| Fat: 3g| Carbohydrates: 5g| Fiber: 1g| Sodium: 50mg| Potassium: 200mg|Phosphorous: 40mg

VEGGIE AND SPROUT RICE PAPER ROLLS

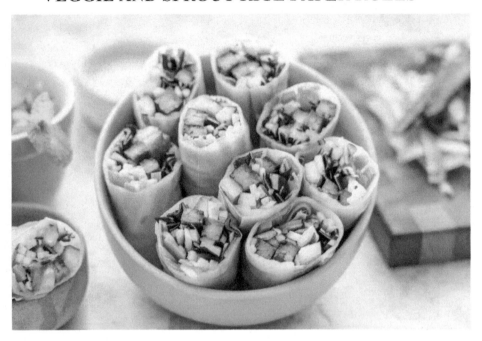

Makes: 2

INGREDIENTS:

☐½ cucumber, cut into matchsticks

☐A handful of bean sprouts

☐Uncooked Rice paper

☐4 spring onions

☐Handful of coriander, chopped

☐1 carrot, cut into matchsticks

☐Liquid Aminos

☐1 chili

INSTRUCTIONS:

a)Soften the rice paper rolls by immersing them in a large bowl of boiling water until they become pliable.

b)Combine the coriander with the remaining ingredients, and place them onto the rice paper wrappers.

c)Roll the wrappers, and then drizzle them with Liquid Aminos for added flavor.

NUTRITION PER SERVING:

Calories: 100-150 kcal | Fat: 2-4 grams | Saturated Fat: 0-1 gram | Sodium: 100-200mg | Carbohydrates: 15-20 grams | Fiber: 2-4 grams | Sugars: 2-4 grams | Protein: 3-5 grams | Phosphorus: 50-100mg | Potassium: 150-200mg

JALAPEÑO POPPER BALLS

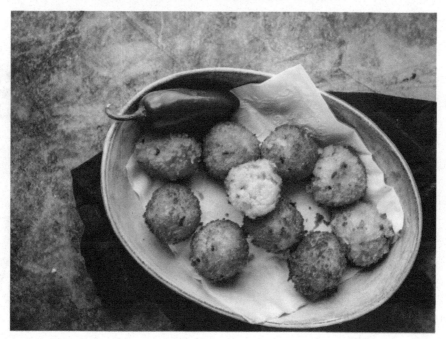

Makes: 2 Servings

INGREDIENTS:
☐¼ teaspoon Onion Powder
☐½ teaspoon Dried Parsley
☐3 ounces of Low-fat Cream Cheese
☐3 slices Turkey Bacon, cooked crisp (lower sodium option)
☐¼ teaspoon Garlic Powder
☐1 Jalapeño Pepper, sliced
☐Salt and Pepper to Taste

INSTRUCTIONS:
a)Mix low-fat cream cheese, jalapeño, spices, salt, and pepper in a bowl until well blended.
b)Gradually add minimal bacon grease or olive oil, stirring until the mixture reaches a firm consistency.
c)Crumble turkey bacon on a platter.
d)Shape the cream cheese mixture into small balls, and roll in crumbled turkey bacon to coat the exterior.

NUTRITION PER SERVING:
Calories: 250 | Protein: 10g | Fat: 15g | Carbohydrates: 10g | Fiber: 2g | Sodium: 450mg | Potassium: 180mg | Phosphorous: 120mg

WHOLE-WHEAT HAM AND CHEESE STROMBOLI

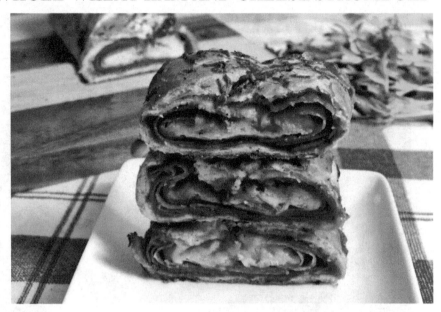

Makes: 2 Servings

INGREDIENTS:

☐1 package (about 12 ounces) of whole wheat pizza dough (choose a lower sodium option if available)

☐4 slices low-sodium ham

☐4 slices low-sodium Swiss cheese

☐½ cup spinach leaves

☐¼ teaspoon garlic powder

☐¼ teaspoon onion powder

☐Black pepper to taste

☐Olive oil spray (or use a small amount of olive oil)

INSTRUCTIONS:

a)Preheat your oven to the temperature specified on the pizza dough package.

b)Roll out the pizza dough on a lightly floured surface into a rectangular shape.

c)Layer the slices of ham, Swiss cheese, and spinach evenly over the rolled-out pizza dough.

d)Sprinkle garlic powder, onion powder, and black pepper over the layers. Roll the dough into a log, enclosing the ham, cheese, and spinach. Place the rolled Stromboli on a baking sheet lined with parchment paper. Lightly spray the top of the Stromboli with olive oil or brush a small amount of olive oil over it.

e)Bake in the preheated oven according to the pizza dough package instructions, or until the crust is golden brown and the cheese is melted. Allow it to cool for a few minutes before slicing.

NUTRITION PER SERVING:

Calories: 400 | Protein: 20g | Fat: 15g | Carbohydrates: 50g | Fiber: 5g | Sodium: 500mg (depending on the pizza dough and ham used) | Potassium: 200mg | Phosphorous: 150mg

MINI PORTOBELLO PIZZAS

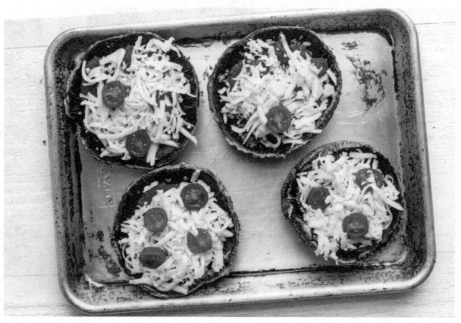

Makes: 2 Servings

INGREDIENTS:

☐4 large Portobello mushroom caps, cleaned and stems removed

☐½ cup low-sodium pizza sauce

☐½ cup shredded low-fat mozzarella cheese

☐¼ cup sliced cherry tomatoes

☐¼ cup sliced black olives (rinse to reduce sodium)

☐¼ cup chopped fresh basil

☐Olive oil spray (or use a small amount of olive oil)

☐Salt and pepper to taste

INSTRUCTIONS:

a)Preheat oven to 375°F (190°C).

b)Lightly spray caps with olive oil, and place on a parchment-lined baking sheet. Bake for 10 minutes.

c)Remove caps from the oven, and drain excess liquid. Spread low-sodium pizza sauce on each cap.

d)Sprinkle shredded low-fat mozzarella evenly over the sauce. Top with sliced cherry tomatoes, black olives, and chopped fresh basil. Season with salt and pepper to taste. Bake mini Portobello pizzas for 10-12 minutes until cheese is melted and bubbly. Allow to cool for a few minutes before serving.

NUTRITION PER SERVING:

Calories: 180 | Protein: 15g | Fat: 8g | Carbohydrates: 15g | Fiber: 5g | Sodium: 200mg (depending on the pizza sauce and olives used) | Potassium: 500mg | Phosphorous: 150mg

RENAL-FRIENDLY TRAIL MIX

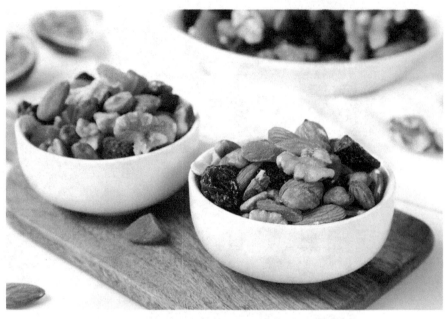

Makes: 2 servings

INGREDIENTS:

☐ ½ cup unsalted almonds

☐ ½ cup unsalted walnuts

☐ ¼ cup pumpkin seeds (pepitas)

☐ ¼ cup sunflower seeds (unsalted)

☐ 2 tablespoons dried cranberries (choose a variety with no added phosphates or potassium)

☐ 2 tablespoons air-popped popcorn (unsalted)

INSTRUCTIONS:

a)In a bowl, combine unsalted almonds, unsalted walnuts, pumpkin seeds, sunflower seeds, dried cranberries, and air-popped popcorn.

b)Toss the ingredients together until well mixed.

c)Portion the trail mix into individual servings for convenient snacking.

NUTRITION PER SERVING:

Calories: Approximately 250 | Protein: 10g | Fat: 20g | Carbohydrates: 15g | Fiber: 5g | Sodium: Minimal (depending on the specific products used) | Potassium: 180mg | Phosphorous: 150mg

ROASTED CHICKPEAS SNACK

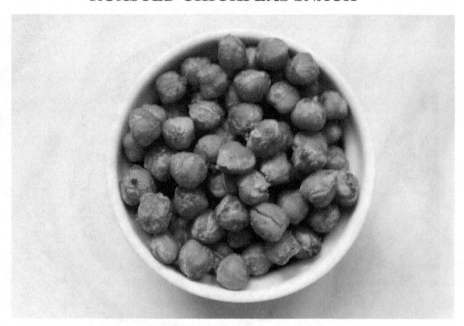

Makes: 2 servings

INGREDIENTS:

☐1 can (15 ounces) low-sodium chickpeas, drained and rinsed

☐1 tablespoon olive oil

☐1 teaspoon ground cumin

☐½ teaspoon paprika

☐¼ teaspoon cayenne pepper (adjust to taste)

☐Salt to taste

INSTRUCTIONS:

a)Preheat the oven to 400°F (200°C).

b)Pat dry the chickpeas with a paper towel and spread them on a baking sheet lined with parchment paper.

c)In a small bowl, mix olive oil, ground cumin, paprika, cayenne pepper, and a pinch of salt.

d)Drizzle the spice mixture over the chickpeas and toss them to coat evenly.

e)Roast the chickpeas in the preheated oven for 25-30 minutes or until they become crispy, shaking the pan occasionally for even cooking. Remove from the oven and let the roasted chickpeas cool.

f)Once cooled, store in an airtight container for a crunchy snack.

NUTRITION PER SERVING:

Calories: Approximately 150 | Protein: 7g | Fat: 7g | Carbohydrates: 17g | Fiber: 5g | Sodium: 20mg | Potassium: Around 180mg | Phosphorous: Around 90mg

EDAMAME AND SEA SALT

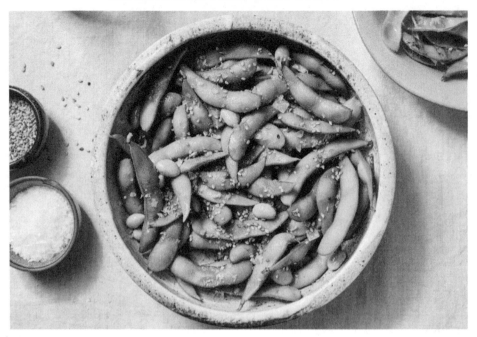

Makes: 1 serving

INGREDIENTS:

☐1 cup edamame, steamed

☐Sea salt to taste

INSTRUCTIONS:

a)Steam edamame according to package instructions.

b)Sprinkle with sea salt to taste.

c)Enjoy this protein-packed and nutritious snack.

NUTRITION PER SERVING:

Calories: Approximately 150 | Protein: 13g | Fat: 9g | Carbohydrates: 8g | Fiber: 4g | Sodium: 5mg | Potassium: Around 400mg | Phosphorous: Around 180mg

PISTACHIO AND DARK CHOCOLATE BARK

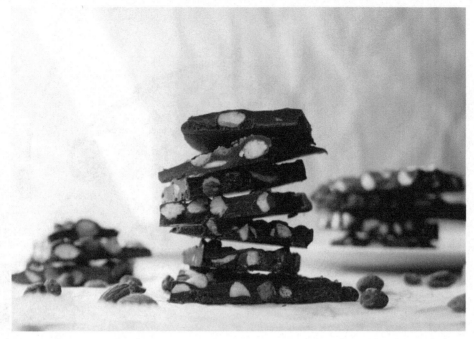

Makes: 1 serving

INGREDIENTS:

☐2 tablespoons shelled pistachios

☐0.9 ounces unsweetened dark chocolate, melted (low phosphorus and potassium content)

☐Pinch of ground cinnamon (optional) instead of sea salt

INSTRUCTIONS:

a)Spread melted dark chocolate on a parchment-lined tray.

b)Evenly distribute shelled pistachios on top of the melted dark chocolate.

c)Optionally, sprinkle a pinch of ground cinnamon for flavor (avoiding extra sodium from sea salt).

d)Refrigerate until the chocolate is set, typically around 1 hour.

e)Once set, break the bark into pieces.

NUTRITION PER SERVING:

Calories: 160 | Protein: 4g | Fat: 12g | Carbohydrates: 14g | Fiber: 3g | Sodium: 5mg (from pistachios, actual sodium content may vary) | Potassium: Around 200mg | Phosphorous: Around 100mg

SWEET POTATO TOAST WITH ALMOND BUTTER AND BERRIES

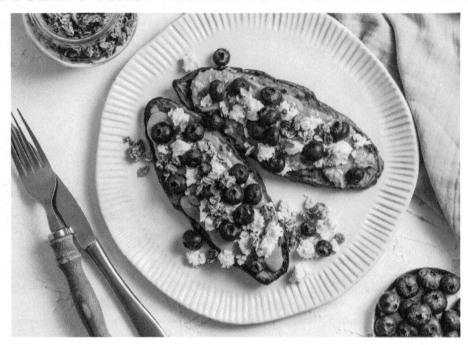

Makes: 1 Serving

INGREDIENTS:

☐½ medium sweet potato, sliced and roasted (ensure portion control based on your dietary needs)

☐2 tablespoons unsalted almond butter

☐Fresh berries (strawberries, blueberries)

INSTRUCTIONS:

a)Roast sweet potato slices until tender. You can do this by placing them in the oven at 400°F (200°C) for about 15-20 minutes or until they are cooked to your liking.

b)Once the sweet potato slices are roasted, let them cool slightly.

c)Spread unsalted almond butter on each sweet potato slice. Ensure portion control, and you can adjust the amount of almond butter based on your preferences.

d)Top with fresh berries, such as strawberries and blueberries.

e)Enjoy this unique and nutritious Sweet Potato Toast!

NUTRITION PER SERVING:

Calories: 250 | Protein: 6g | Fat: 15g | Carbohydrates: 25g | Fiber: 6g | Sodium: 30mg (from sweet potatoes, actual sodium content may vary) | Potassium: Around 300mg | Phosphorous: Around 100mg

DATE AND PISTACHIO BITES

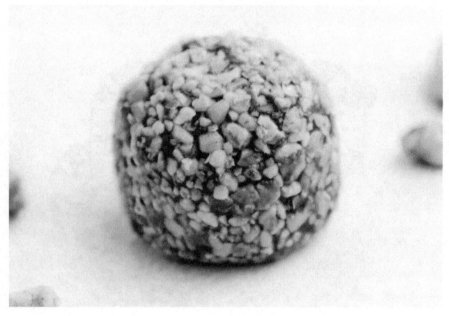

Makes: 1 serving

INGREDIENTS:

☐3 Medjool dates, pitted

☐2 tablespoons unsalted pistachios, finely chopped

☐2 teaspoons low-fat cream cheese or goat cheese

☐½ teaspoon honey

☐¼ teaspoon ground cumin

☐⅛ teaspoon ground paprika

☐Pinch of salt

☐Pinch of black pepper

☐Fresh parsley leaves for garnish (optional)

INSTRUCTIONS:

a)Pulse unsalted pistachios in a food processor until finely chopped. Transfer to a shallow bowl.

b)In the same processor, blend low-fat cream cheese (or goat cheese), honey, cumin, paprika, salt, and black pepper until smooth. Carefully open each pitted date to create a small pocket.

c)Stuff each date with about ½ teaspoon of the cheese mixture.

d)Roll stuffed dates in chopped pistachios, ensuring they adhere to the cheese mixture.

e)Place on a serving platter. Optionally, garnish with fresh parsley leaves. Serve immediately.

NUTRITION PER SERVING:

Calories: 180 | Protein: 3g | Fat: 7g | Carbohydrates: 30g | Fiber: 3g | Sodium: 30mg (actual sodium content may vary) | Potassium: Around 300mg | Phosphorous: Around 60mg

DARK CHOCOLATE ALMOND BITES

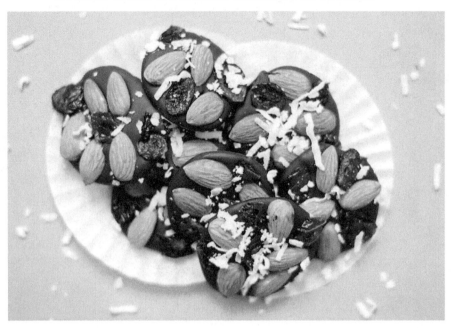

Makes: 1 Serving

INGREDIENTS:

☐2 tablespoons unsalted almond butter

☐1 tablespoon honey

☐1 tablespoon coconut oil (use a minimal amount)

☐1 tablespoon unsweetened cocoa powder

☐¼ teaspoon vanilla extract

☐A pinch of salt

☐Sliced almonds for garnish (optional)

INSTRUCTIONS:

a)In a saucepan, combine unsalted almond butter, honey, and a minimal amount of coconut oil over low heat. Stir until well combined.

b)Remove from heat and stir in the unsweetened cocoa powder, vanilla extract, and a pinch of salt.

c)Pour the mixture into a small container lined with parchment paper.

d)Sprinkle sliced almonds on top for added texture, if desired.

e)Refrigerate for about 1-2 hours, or until the mixture is set.

f)Once set, use the parchment paper to lift the mixture out of the container. Cut into bite-sized squares or rectangles.

NUTRITION PER SERVING:

Calories: 220 | Protein: 4g | Fat: 15g | Carbohydrates: 18g | Fiber: 3g | Sodium: 10mg (actual sodium content may vary) | Potassium: Around 180mg | Phosphorous: Around 80mg

CUCUMBER AND SMOKED SALMON BITES

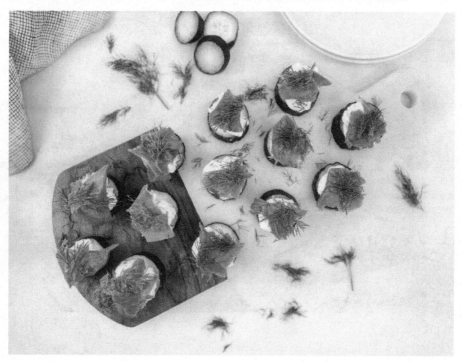

Makes: 1 serving

INGREDIENTS:

☐1 cucumber, cut into rounds

☐2 ounces smoked salmon (choose a brand with lower sodium content)

☐2 tablespoons dairy-free cream cheese or cashew cheese

☐Fresh dill for garnish

INSTRUCTIONS:

a)Arrange the cucumber rounds on a serving platter.

b)Place a small amount (about ½ teaspoon) of dairy-free cream cheese or cashew cheese on each cucumber round. Top each cucumber round with a piece of smoked salmon.

c)Garnish with fresh dill on top for added flavor.

d)Serve immediately and enjoy these refreshing and kidney-friendly bites!

NUTRITION PER SERVING:

Calories: 150 | Protein: 12g | Fat: 8g | Carbohydrates: 8g | Fiber: 2g | Sodium: 250mg (actual sodium content may vary) | Potassium: Around 300mg | Phosphorous: Around 150mg

PUMPKIN TAHINI AND CASHEW DIP

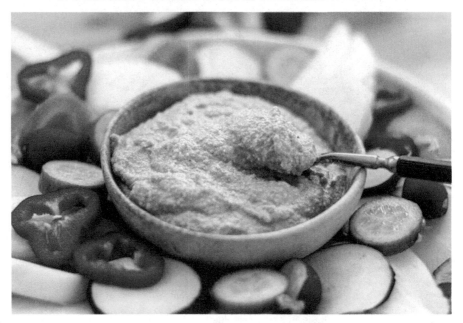

Makes: 1 serving

INGREDIENTS:

☐¼ cup canned pumpkin puree with no additives

☐1 tablespoon tahini

☐1 tablespoon unsalted cashews

☐1 clove garlic, minced

☐½ tablespoon fresh lemon juice

☐½ teaspoon olive oil

☐⅛ teaspoon ground cumin

☐Pinch of ground paprika

☐Salt and pepper to taste

☐Optional garnish: extra unsalted cashews, and a sprinkle of paprika

INSTRUCTIONS:

a)In a food processor, combine canned pumpkin, tahini, unsalted cashews, minced garlic, lemon juice, olive oil, ground cumin, ground paprika, salt, and pepper. Blend until smooth and creamy, scraping down the sides as needed. Taste and adjust seasonings, adding more salt, pepper, or lemon juice if necessary.

b)Transfer to a serving dish. Optionally, garnish with extra cashews and a sprinkle of paprika.

c)Serve with fresh vegetable sticks or paleo-friendly crackers.

NUTRITION PER SERVING:

Calories: 150 | Protein: 4g | Fat: 10g | Carbohydrates: 14g | Fiber: 3g | Sodium: 20mg (actual sodium content may vary) | Potassium: Around 200mg | Phosphorous: Around 80mg

BAKED APPLE WITH CINNAMON

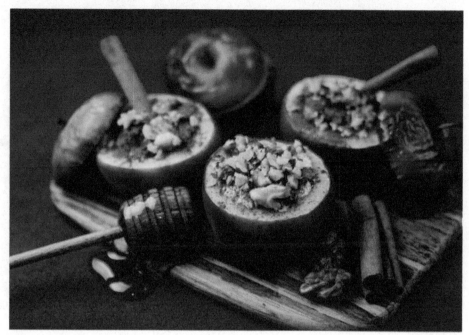

Makes: 1 serving

INGREDIENTS:

☐1 apple (any variety)

☐½ teaspoon cinnamon

☐½ tablespoon honey (optional)

☐1 tablespoon chopped unsalted nuts (e.g., walnuts, almonds)

☐1 tablespoon raisins

INSTRUCTIONS:

a)Preheat your oven to 375°F (190°C).

b)Wash and core the apple, removing the center seeds to create a well in the center.

c)Sprinkle cinnamon evenly inside the apple and drizzle with honey (if desired).

d)Place the apple in a baking dish and add a little water to the bottom of the dish to prevent sticking.

e)Bake in the oven for about 25-30 minutes or until the apple is tender.

f)Sprinkle with chopped unsalted nuts and raisins before serving.

NUTRITION PER SERVING:

Calories: 150 | Protein: 2g | Fat: 7g | Carbohydrates: 26g | Fiber: 4g | Sodium: 5mg (actual sodium content may vary) | Potassium: Around 200mg | Phosphorous: Around 40mg

BAKED ZUCCHINI CHIPS

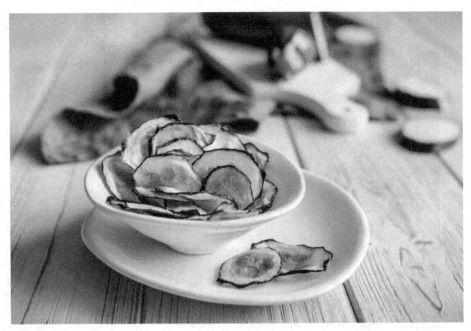

Makes: 1 serving

INGREDIENTS:

☐2 medium zucchinis, thinly sliced

☐1 tablespoon olive oil

☐½ teaspoon garlic powder

☐½ teaspoon onion powder

☐¼ teaspoon dried oregano

☐Salt and pepper to taste

INSTRUCTIONS:

a)Preheat the oven to 375°F (190°C).

b)In a bowl, toss thinly sliced zucchini with olive oil, garlic powder, onion powder, dried oregano, salt, and pepper. Arrange the zucchini slices on a baking sheet lined with parchment paper.

c)Bake for 15-20 minutes or until the zucchini chips are golden and crispy.

d)Allow them to cool slightly before serving.

NUTRITION PER SERVING:

Calories: 80 | Protein: 2g | Fat: 6g | Carbohydrates: 6g | Fiber: 2g | Sodium: 10mg (actual sodium content may vary) | Potassium: 280mg | Phosphorous: 40mg

EGGPLANT AND TOMATO BRUSCHETTA

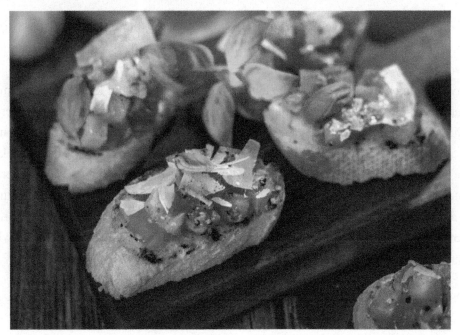

Makes: 2 Servings

INGREDIENTS:
☐1 small eggplant, diced
☐2 tomatoes, diced
☐2 cloves garlic, minced
☐1 tablespoon olive oil
☐1 tablespoon balsamic vinegar
☐1 teaspoon dried oregano
☐Salt and pepper to taste
☐Basil leaves, to garnish
☐Whole grain baguette slices for serving

INSTRUCTIONS:
a)Preheat the oven to 375°F (190°C).
b)Toss diced eggplant, tomatoes, and minced garlic with olive oil, balsamic vinegar, dried oregano, salt, and pepper. Spread the mixture on a baking sheet and roast for 20-25 minutes or until the vegetables are tender.
c)Allow it to cool slightly before serving.
d)Serve the eggplant and tomato mixture on whole-grain baguette slices and garnish with basil leaves.

NUTRITION PER SERVING:
Calories: 120 | Protein: 3g | Fat: 5g | Carbohydrates: 18g | Fiber: 5g | Sodium: 80mg (actual sodium content may vary) | Potassium: 300mg | Phosphorous: 80mg

CHAPTER 3: MAIN COURSE

Welcome to Chapter 3 where we embark on a culinary journey through the heartiest offerings in the Main Course section. These recipes are carefully curated to not only tantalize your taste buds but also prioritize the well-being of your kidneys. From the comforting embrace of Farfalle Pasta with Mushrooms to the zesty allure of Lemon and Thyme Salmon, this chapter is a celebration of wholesome and kidney-friendly main dishes. Indulge in the succulent flavors of Ginger Lemon Tilapia, the savory delights of Roasted Lemon Herb Chicken, and the seafood symphony of Prawns with Asparagus. Each recipe is a testament to the belief that maintaining renal health can be a flavorsome adventure. Whether you're in the mood for a nourishing Chicken and Mushroom Casserole or a vibrant Coral Lentil and Swiss Chard Soup, these main course options offer a diverse array of choices that cater to various tastes and dietary needs. Join us as we explore the richness of Cauliflower Fried Rice with Chicken, the heartiness of Lentil and Butternut Squash Stew, and the exotic notes of Shrimp Curry. Chapter 3 is an invitation to savor the pleasure of a well-rounded and kidney-conscious main course, where every dish is a step toward nourishing your kidneys without compromising on culinary delight.

FARFALLE PASTA WITH MUSHROOMS

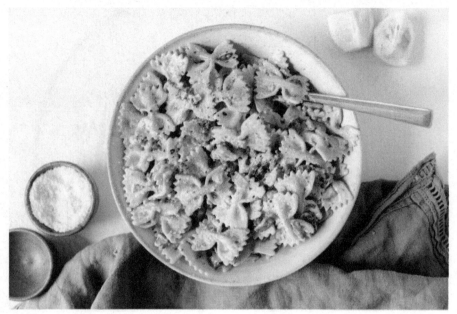

Makes: 4 Servings

INGREDIENTS:

☐1 pound farfalle pasta, cooked

☐Pinch Low-Sodium Salt and pepper to taste

☐2 zucchinis, quartered and sliced

☐8-ounce package of mushrooms, sliced

☐⅓ cup olive oil

☐1 clove of garlic, chopped

☐1 tablespoon paprika

☐1 tablespoon dried oregano

☐¼ cup butter

☐1 onion, chopped

☐1 tomato, chopped

INSTRUCTIONS:

a)In a skillet, heat olive oil and sauté garlic, mushrooms, onion, and tomato for 17 minutes.

b)Season the mixture with salt, pepper, paprika, and oregano to enhance the flavors.

c)Transfer the cooked vegetables to a mixing bowl and combine them with the noodles.

NUTRITION PER SERVING:

Calories: 400 | Protein: 12 grams | Fat: 8 grams | Carbohydrates: 70 grams | Fiber: 5 grams | Sodium: 400mg | Potassium: 500mg | Phosphorus: 200mg

GINGER LEMON TILAPIA

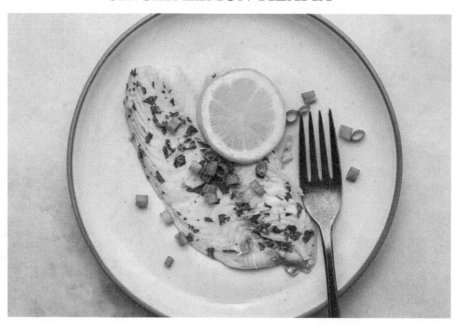

Makes: 4 servings

INGREDIENTS:
- 4 tilapia fillets (about 6 ounces each)
- 2 tablespoons olive oil
- 2 tablespoons fresh ginger, grated
- 4 cloves garlic, minced
- Zest and juice of 2 lemons
- 1 teaspoon ground black pepper
- ½ teaspoon salt (or to taste)
- ¼ cup fresh parsley, chopped (for garnish)

INSTRUCTIONS:
a)Preheat the oven to 400°F (200°C).

b)Place tilapia fillets in a baking dish.

c)In a small bowl, mix olive oil, grated ginger, minced garlic, lemon zest, lemon juice, black pepper, and salt.

d)Pour the ginger-lemon mixture over the tilapia fillets, ensuring they are evenly coated.

e)Bake in the preheated oven for 15-20 minutes or until the tilapia is cooked through and flakes easily with a fork. Garnish with chopped fresh parsley before serving.

NUTRITION PER SERVING:
Calories: 230 | Protein: 26g | Fat: 12g | Carbohydrates: 3g | Fiber: 1g | Sodium: Sodium content may vary based on ingredients; choose low-sodium options when available. | Potassium: 300mg | Phosphorous: 220mg

LEMON AND THYME SALMON

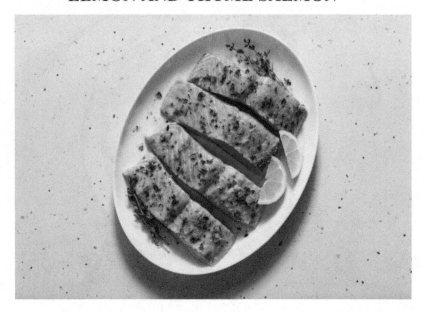

Makes: 4

INGREDIENTS:

☐1 lemon, sliced thin

☐1 tablespoon fresh thyme

☐32 ounces piece of salmon

☐1 tablespoons capers

☐Pinch low Sodium salt and freshly ground pepper

☐Olive oil

INSTRUCTIONS:

a)Preheat your oven to 400 degrees Fahrenheit and line a rimmed baking sheet with parchment paper.

b)Place the salmon fillets, skin side down, on the prepared baking sheet.

c)Season the salmon with salt and pepper, ensuring it is evenly coated.

d)Scatter capers over the salmon, evenly distribute sliced lemon on top, and sprinkle fresh thyme leaves over the fillets. Place the baking sheet in the preheated oven and bake for approximately 25 minutes, or until the salmon is cooked through and flakes easily with a fork.

e)Once cooked, remove from the oven and let the salmon rest for a few minutes before serving.

NUTRITION PER SERVING:

Calories: 330 | Fat 17.7g | Saturated fat 2.6g | Polyunsaturated fat 5.6 | Cholesterol 109.1mg | Sodium 126.5mg | Carbohydrates 1g | Sugar 0g | Fiber 0.4g | Protein 39.5g | Phosphorus: 300-400mg | Potassium: 400-600mg

COD IN TOMATO SAUCE

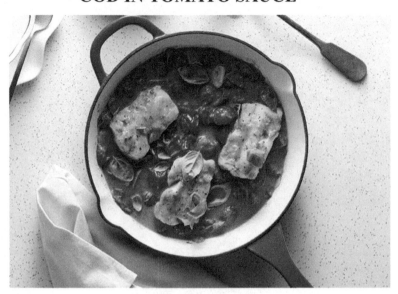

Makes: 4 servings

INGREDIENTS:

☐ 3 tablespoons Light Olive Oil

☐ 4 pieces Fresh Cod Fillets (approximately 7-9 ounces each)

☐ 10.5 ounces Cherry Tomatoes, cut in half

☐ ¼ cup Garlic, chopped finely

☐ ½ cup Chardonnay White Wine

☐ Juice of 1 Lemon

☐ Salt and Pepper to taste

INSTRUCTIONS:

a)Heat oil in a large sauté pan. Season the cod fillets with a minimal amount of salt and pepper. Fry the fish until lightly golden and tender, approximately 3 minutes on each side. Remove from the pan and set aside.

b)Using the same pan, sauté the cherry tomatoes until they are soft and blistering. Add more oil if the pan starts to dry up. Add the chopped garlic and sauté for about a minute.

c)Pour in the white wine and let it reduce by half on low heat, about 3-5 minutes. Stir in the lemon juice.

d)Season with a small amount of salt and pepper and stir for a few seconds. Place the fillets back into the pan and simmer for 2 minutes. Transfer cod to a serving dish and pour over the wine tomato sauce.

NUTRITION PER SERVING:

Calories: 350 | Protein: 30g | Fat: 15g | Carbohydrates: 10g | Fiber: 2g | Sodium: 120mg (actual sodium content may vary) | Potassium: 600mg | Phosphorous: 250mg

LEMON PRAWNS

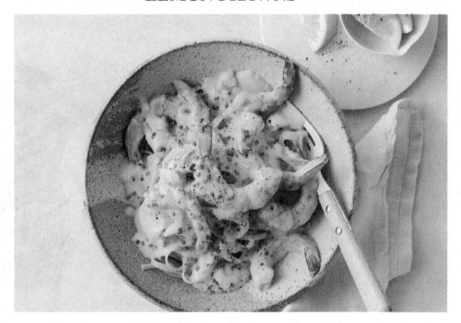

Makes: 6

INGREDIENTS:

- 1 onion, diced
- 1 tablespoon fresh ginger, chopped
- 3 garlic cloves, crushed
- 1 tablespoon fresh lemon zest, finely grated
- 1 fresh red pepper, seeded and chopped
- 1 teaspoon ground turmeric
- ½ cup olive oil
- ½ cup fresh lemon juice
- 20-24 raw shrimp, peeled and deveined
- 1 tablespoon almond oil

INSTRUCTIONS:

a)In a bowl, mix all the ingredients except for the shrimp and almond oil. Add the shrimp to the mixture and generously brush them with the marinade.Cover the bowl and let the shrimp marinate in the refrigerator overnight. Heat the almond oil in a non-stick skillet over high heat and sauté the shrimp for 3 minutes.

b)Pour the reserved marinade into the skillet and bring it to a boil, stirring occasionally.

c)Cook the shrimp in the boiling marinade for approximately 1-2 minutes.

NUTRITION PER SERVING:

Calories: 268 | Fat: 20.6g | Carbohydrates: 4.2g | Fiber: 0.6g | Sugars: 1g | Protein: 17.2g | Sodium: 94.4mg | Phosphorus: 250-350mg | Potassium: 200-300mg

ROASTED LEMON HERB CHICKEN

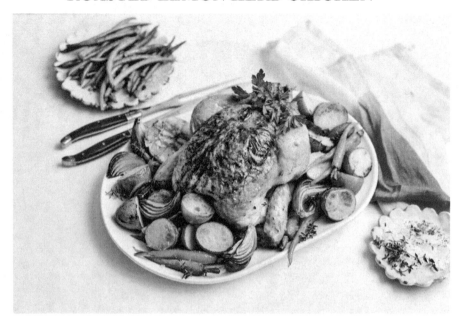

Makes: 4 Servings

INGREDIENTS:

4 bone-in, skin-on chicken thighs

1 lemon, sliced

3 cloves garlic, minced

2 tablespoons fresh rosemary, chopped

2 tablespoons fresh thyme, chopped

2 tablespoons olive oil

Salt, to taste

Pepper, to taste

INSTRUCTIONS:

a) Preheat the oven to 400°F (200°C).

b) In a small bowl, mix together minced garlic, chopped rosemary, chopped thyme, olive oil, salt, and pepper to create a herb marinade. Pat the chicken thighs dry with a paper towel. Rub the herb marinade over each chicken thigh, ensuring they are well coated. Place the chicken thighs in a roasting pan, skin side up.

c) Arrange lemon slices around the chicken pieces. Roast in the preheated oven for 35-40 minutes or until the chicken reaches an internal temperature of 165°F (74°C) and the skin is golden and crispy.

NUTRITION PER SERVING:

Calories: 405.3 | Protein: 32.2g | Carbohydrates: 3.6g | Dietary Fiber: 1.5g | Sugars: 0.1g | Fat: 29.2g | Saturated Fat: 7.8g | Cholesterol: 127.7mg | Sodium: 177.6mg | Phosphorus: 250-350mg | Potassium: 300-400mg

ASPARAGUS AND ZUCCHINI CARBONARA

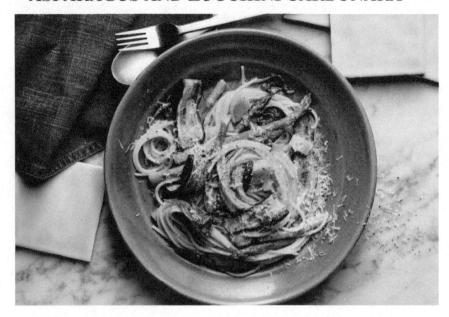

Makes: 4

INGREDIENTS:

☐¼ cup extra virgin olive oil

☐3.5 tablespoons salted butter, chopped

☐2 small zucchini, sliced lengthways

☐2 bunches of asparagus, woody ends trimmed

☐1 large leek, white part only, thickly sliced

☐6 garlic cloves, thinly sliced

☐1.8 ounces baby spinach leaves

☐1.1 pounds low phosphorus and low sodium spaghetti, cooked until al dente

☐4 large egg yolks, at room temperature (reserve egg whites for another use)

☐1 cup very finely grated parmesan (choose a low-sodium variety), plus extra to serve

☐Finely grated zest and juice of 1 small lemon

INSTRUCTIONS:

a)Heat oil and butter in a large frypan. Cook zucchini until golden, then transfer to a plate and cover.

b)Cook asparagus until tender and golden; transfer to the plate with zucchini.

c)Cook leek and garlic, then add spinach until wilted. Return zucchini and asparagus to the pan.

d)Whisk yolks, parmesan, and cold water. Transfer pasta to the frypan, and toss with vegetables. Temper egg yolk mixture, pour over pasta, and toss. Add lemon zest and juice, season, and serve with extra parmesan.

NUTRITION PER SERVING:

Calories: 650 | Protein: 24g | Fat: 27g | Carbohydrates: 77g | Fiber: 4g | Sodium: 350mg (actual sodium content may vary) | Potassium: 400mg | Phosphorous: 250mg

PRAWNS WITH ASPARAGUS

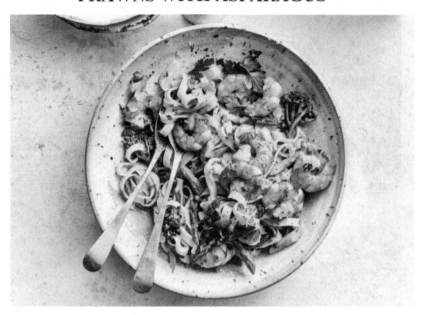

Makes: 4

INGREDIENTS:

☐1 bunch of asparagus, peeled and chopped

☐1-pound shrimp, peeled and deveined

☐⅔ cup chicken broth

☐4 garlic cloves, crushed

☐½ teaspoon ground ginger

☐2 tablespoons fresh lemon juice

☐2 tablespoons almond oil

INSTRUCTIONS:

a)Heat the almond oil in a skillet over medium heat until melted.

b)Put all the ingredients (excluding the broth) into the skillet and cook for approximately 2 minutes.

c)Stir the mixture and continue cooking for around 5 minutes.

d)Incorporate the broth into the skillet and cook for approximately 2 to 4 minutes.

NUTRITION PER SERVING:

Calories: 241 | Fat: 9.2g | Carbohydrates: 9.8g | Fiber: 3.7g | Sugars: 3.5 g | Protein: 30.7g | Sodium: 250mg | Phosphorus: 200-300mg | Potassium: 400-600mg

SEA BASS WITH VEGETABLES

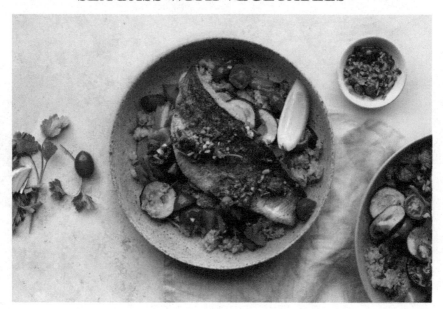

Makes: 2 Servings

INGREDIENTS:
☐1 sea bass fillet, diced

☐¼ teaspoon ginger paste

☐¼ teaspoon garlic paste

☐1 tablespoon coconut vinegar

☐Pinch of salt

☐1 tablespoon olive oil, extra-virgin

☐½ cup fresh button mushrooms, sliced

☐1 small onion, quartered

☐1/2 cup mixed bell peppers, seeded and diced

INSTRUCTIONS:
a)In a bowl, marinate the sea bass with ginger paste, garlic paste, coconut vinegar, and salt for 10 minutes.

b)Heat olive oil in a pan over medium heat. Add marinated sea bass and cook until golden brown. Set aside. Add mushrooms, onions, and bell peppers. Sauté until vegetables are tender yet crisp.

c)Serve the Sea Bass with Vegetables hot.

NUTRITION PER SERVING:
Calories: 280 | Fat: 17.6g | Carbs: 8.8g | Fiber: 2.2g | Sugars: 3.8g | Protein: 23.9g | Sodium: 200-400mg | Phosphorus: 250-350mg | Potassium: 400-600mg

CHICKEN AND MUSHROOM CASSEROLE

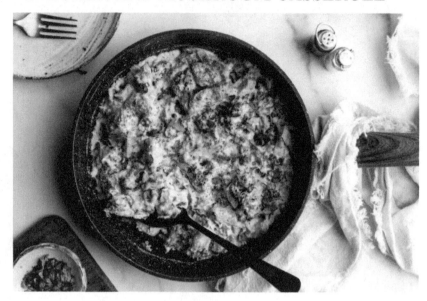

Makes: 4

INGREDIENTS:

☐⅓ cup Dijon mustard

☐⅓ cup raw honey

☐1 teaspoon basil (dried)

☐4 breasts of chicken

☐¼ teaspoon ground turmeric

☐1 cup fresh button mushrooms, sliced

☐1 teaspoon crumbled dried basil

☐Pinch Low-Sodium Salt

☐Pinch black pepper, ground

☐½ head of broccoli, cut into florets

INSTRUCTIONS:

a)Preheat the oven to 350ºF and grease a baking dish.

b)Combine all the ingredients, excluding the chicken, mushrooms, and broccoli, in a mixing bowl.

c)Arrange the chicken, broccoli florets, and mushrooms in the greased casserole dish. Evenly spoon half of the honey mixture over the chicken and broccoli. Place the dish in the oven and bake for about 20 minutes.

d)Take the dish out of the oven, baste the remaining sauce over the chicken, and continue baking for another 10 minutes.

NUTRITION PER SERVING:

Calories: 386 | Fat: 11.5g | Carbohydrates: 27.4g | Fiber: 1.9g | Sugars: 24.3g | Protein: 43.6g | Sodium 174 mg | Phosphorus: 300-400mg | Potassium: 400-600mg

CAULIFLOWER FRIED RICE WITH CHICKEN

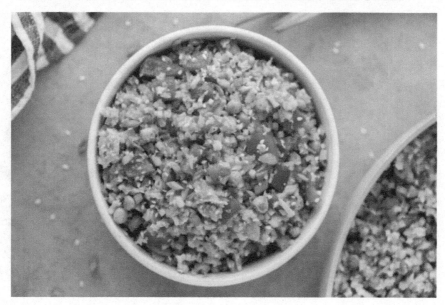

Makes: 4 servings

INGREDIENTS:

☐1 small head of cauliflower

☐2 tablespoons sesame oil (choose a lower sodium option, if available)

☐1 small white onion, chopped

☐1 ½ cups low-sodium frozen peas and carrots

☐2 cloves garlic, minced

☐2 large eggs

☐1 ½ cups shredded or diced cooked chicken (cooked without added phosphorus-based seasonings)

☐¼ cup low-sodium soy sauce, plus extra for serving (or use tamari or coconut aminos)

INSTRUCTIONS:

a)Rinse and pat cauliflower dry, cut into chunks, and pulse in a food processor until it resembles rice.

b)Heat sesame oil in a large skillet over medium heat. Sauté onion for 3-4 minutes until softened.

c)Add frozen peas, carrots, and garlic, and stir until tender, about 2-3 minutes.

d)Crack eggs into the pan, and stir until scrambled and mixed with vegetables.

e)Add chicken, cauliflower rice, and low-sodium soy sauce.

f)Stir until well combined and heated through, about 2-3 minutes.

g)Serve with extra low-sodium soy sauce if desired.

NUTRITION PER SERVING:

Calories: 250 | Protein: 20g | Fat: 10g | Carbohydrates: 18g | Fiber: 6g | Sodium: 300mg (adjusted for lower-sodium options) | Potassium: 400mg | Phosphorous: 200mg

CORAL LENTIL AND SWISS CHARD SOUP

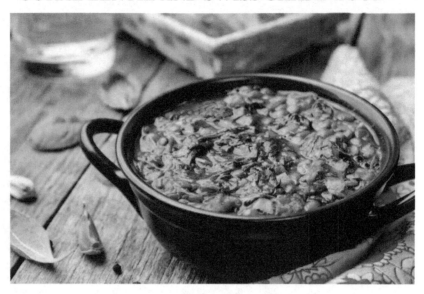

Makes: 4

INGREDIENTS:

☐2 tablespoons olive oil

☐1 medium onion, diced

☐2 carrots, diced

☐½ teaspoon ginger powder

☐2 minced big garlic cloves

☐1 teaspoon cumin powder

☐½ teaspoon red pepper flakes

☐½ teaspoons low sodium salt

☐15-ounce can of diced tomatoes

☐1 cup dried red lentils

☐8 cups of vegetable broth

☐1 bunch of Swiss chard, coarsely chopped

INSTRUCTIONS:

a)Heat oil in a soup or casserole dish. Sauté onion and carrot for 7 minutes.

b)Add garlic, cumin, ginger, chili flakes, and salt to the dish. Stir in tomatoes and cook for 5 minutes.

c)Add lentils and broth, bringing it to a boil. Then, reduce the heat to low and let it cook uncovered for 10 minutes until the lentils are tender. Continue cooking for another 5 minutes until the chard has wilted.

d)Season with salt and pepper according to your taste. Serve with a wedge of lemon for added flavor.

NUTRITION PER SERVING:

Calories: 370 | Fat 9g | Saturated fat 5g | Carbohydrate 57g | Dietary fiber 25g | Protein 20g | Sodium 90.67mg | Potassium: 150mg | Phosphorus: 50mg

TOFU AND SPINACH LASAGNE

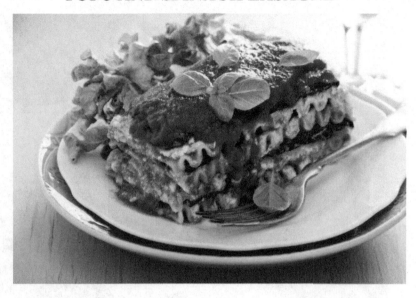

Makes: 2

INGREDIENTS:

☐6 lasagna noodles (cooked according to package instructions, choose a lower sodium option)

☐1 tablespoon olive oil

☐1 medium onion, finely chopped

☐2 cloves garlic, minced

☐8 ounces firm tofu, drained and crumbled

☐2 cups fresh spinach, chopped

☐1 can (14 ounces) diced tomatoes, no salt added

☐1 can (6 ounces) tomato paste, no salt added

☐1 teaspoon each of dried basil, oregano, and salt and pepper to taste

☐½ cup low-fat mozzarella cheese, shredded

☐Fresh basil leaves for garnish (optional)

INSTRUCTIONS:

a)In a large skillet, heat olive oil over medium heat. Sauté chopped onion until softened, then add minced garlic and sauté for an additional minute. Add crumbled tofu, and cook for 5 minutes, stirring occasionally.

b)Stir in chopped spinach, and cook until wilted. Add diced tomatoes, tomato paste, dried basil, dried oregano, salt, and pepper. Simmer for about 10 minutes.

c)In a baking dish, layer three lasagna noodles, half of the tofu-spinach mixture, and half of the mozzarella cheese. Repeat layers. Bake at 375° for 30 minutes or until bubbly. Garnish with fresh basil.

NUTRITION PER SERVING:

Calories: 400 | Protein: 20g | Fat: 12g | Carbohydrates: 50g | Fiber: 8g | Sodium: 200mg (adjusted for lower-sodium options) | Potassium: 300mg | Phosphorous: 150mg

LENTIL AND BUTTERNUT SQUASH STEW

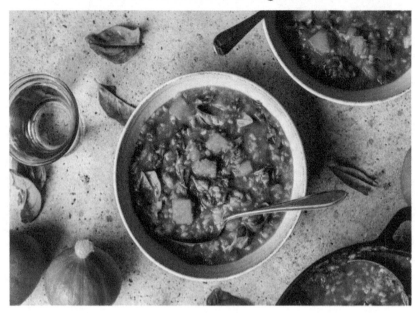

Makes: 4

INGREDIENTS:

☐225g brown lentils, soaked

☐2 brown onions

☐750ml wheat-free vegetable stock

☐4 carrots

☐½ butternut squash

☐1 sweet potato

☐2 white potatoes

☐1 stick of celery

☐A handful of fresh garden peas

☐Handful watercress

☐2 tablespoons fresh dill

☐1 teaspoon tamari sauce

INSTRUCTIONS:

a)In a pan, bring the stock and onions to a boil.

b)Add lentils, potatoes, squash, and carrots to the pan and let it simmer for 15 minutes.

c)Include the celery, fresh peas, leaves, and dill into the mixture.

NUTRITION PER SERVING:

195 Calories: | Protein 7.8g | Carbohydrates 24.2g | Fiber 3.7g | Sugar 2.1 g | Fat 8.3g | Saturated fat 4.3g | Sodium: 300mg | Potassium: 450mg | Phosphorus: 150mg

SHRIMP CURRY

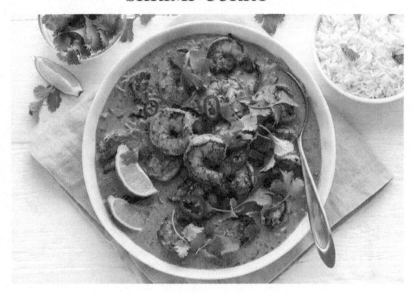

Makes: 4 servings

INGREDIENTS:

☐ 1 pound shrimp, peeled and deveined

☐ 1 tablespoon olive oil

☐ 1 onion, finely chopped

☐ 2 cloves garlic, minced

☐ 1 tablespoon curry powder

☐ 1 teaspoon turmeric

☐ 1 teaspoon cumin

☐ 1 can (14 ounces) low-sodium diced tomatoes, undrained

☐ 1 can (14 ounces) coconut milk

☐ Low-sodium salt and pepper to taste

☐ Fresh cilantro for garnish

INSTRUCTIONS:

a) In a large skillet, heat olive oil over medium heat. Sauté chopped onions until translucent.

b) Add minced garlic to the skillet, and cook for an additional minute. Stir in curry powder, turmeric, and cumin; cook for 2-3 minutes until spices are fragrant. Add low-sodium diced tomatoes with their juice to the skillet. Simmer for 5 minutes. Pour in coconut milk and bring the mixture to a gentle simmer.

f) Add shrimp to the skillet, cook until opaque and cooked through (5-7 minutes). Season curry with low-sodium salt and pepper to taste. Serve over steamed rice or cauliflower rice. Garnish with cilantro.

NUTRITION PER SERVING:

Calories: 300 | Protein: 25g | Fat: 20g | Carbohydrates: 10g | Fiber: 3g | Sodium: 200mg | Potassium: 500mg | Phosphorous: 200mg

LEFTOVER TURKEY TACO SALAD

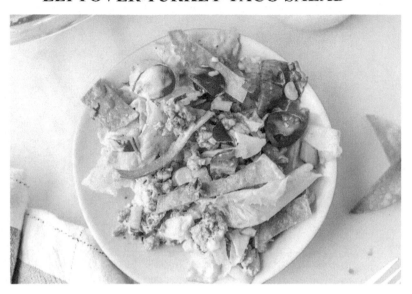

Makes: 4 servings

INGREDIENTS:

☐4 cups mixed salad greens (lettuce, spinach, or your choice)

☐2 cups leftover turkey, shredded or diced

☐1 cup cherry tomatoes, halved

☐1 cup low-potassium black beans, drained and rinsed

☐1 cup low-potassium corn kernels (fresh, canned, or frozen)

☐½ red onion, thinly sliced

☐½ cup shredded low-phosphorus cheddar cheese

☐1 small avocado, sliced

☐2 tablespoons olive oil

☐1 teaspoon low-sodium taco seasoning

INSTRUCTIONS:

a)Combine greens, turkey, cherry tomatoes, black beans, corn, red onion, and cheddar cheese in a bowl.

b)In a small bowl, whisk together the olive oil, and low-sodium taco seasoning to create the dressing. Drizzle the dressing over the salad and toss gently to combine. Top the salad with sliced avocado.

NUTRITION PER SERVING:

Calories: 300| Protein: 20g| Fat: 15g|Carbohydrates: 25g| Fiber: 7g| Sodium: 200mg| Potassium: 350mg| Phosphorus: 150mg

SPINACH, SHRIMP, AND TANGERINE BOWL

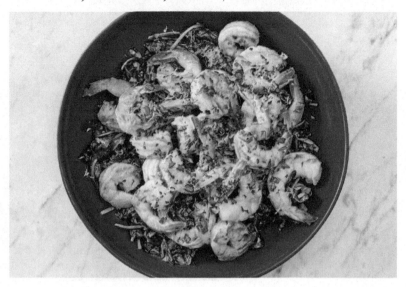

Makes: 4 Servings

INGREDIENTS:

☐ 1 cup endive

☐ 1 tablespoon parsley, chopped

☐ 1/4 small red onion, sliced into rings

☐ 3 cups spinach

☐ 1 tablespoon clarified butter

☐ 1/2 cup cooked shrimp (tails removed)

☐ 2 small tangerines, peeled and sectioned

☐ 1/4 cup roasted pine nuts

☐ 1 tablespoon basil, chopped

☐ 1 teaspoon fresh lime juice

INSTRUCTIONS:

a) Combine the chopped onion, spinach, endive, basil, and parsley. Mix them to evenly distribute the ingredients. Heat butter in a skillet over medium heat. Add the shrimp and lime juice to the skillet and cook for about one minute, stirring occasionally, until the shrimp are cooked through and opaque. Remove shrimp from the skillet and add them to the salad bowl with the other ingredients. Sprinkle pine nuts over the salad.

b) Drizzle your choice of dressing over the salad and toss everything together to coat the ingredients evenly with the dressing. Plate the salad and garnish with tangerine wedges.

NUTRITION PER SERVING:

Calories: 239 | Fat 22g (Saturated 5g) | Cholesterol 35mg | Sodium 48mg | Carbohydrate 7g | Dietary Fiber 2g | Protein 7g | Phosphorus: 250-350mg | Potassium: 500-700mg

CHICKEN AND SPINACH PASTA SALAD

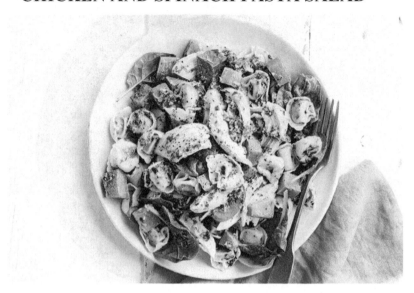

Makes: 4 servings

INGREDIENTS:

□8 ounces spinach and ricotta tortellini (choose a lower sodium option)

□1 cup cooked and shredded chicken breast (cooked without added phosphorus-based seasonings)

□1 cup fresh spinach, chopped

□½ cup cooked pumpkin, diced

□2 tablespoons homemade or store-bought low-phosphorus pesto

□2 tablespoons extra-virgin olive oil

□1 tablespoon balsamic vinegar (low sodium)

□Salt and pepper to taste

□Fresh basil leaves for garnish (optional)

INSTRUCTIONS:

a)Cook the spinach and ricotta tortellini according to the package instructions. Drain and let it cool.

b)In a large mixing bowl, combine the cooked and shredded chicken, chopped fresh spinach, and diced cooked pumpkin. Add the cooled spinach and ricotta tortellini to the bowl.

c)In a separate small bowl, whisk together the low-phosphorus pesto, extra-virgin olive oil, and balsamic vinegar. Pour the pesto dressing over the pasta salad and toss gently to combine.

d)Season with salt and pepper to taste. Garnish with fresh basil leaves if desired.

e)Chill the pasta salad in the refrigerator for at least 30 minutes before serving.

NUTRITION PER SERVING:

Calories: 350 | Protein: 20g | Fat: 15g | Carbohydrates: 30g | Fiber: 5g | Sodium: 150mg (adjusted for lower-sodium options) | Potassium: 300mg | Phosphorous: 150mg

SALMON FETTUCCINI

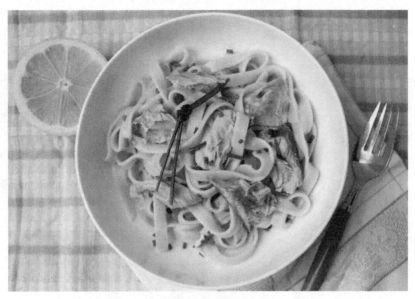

Makes: 6 Servings

INGREDIENTS:

☐12 ounces fresh salmon, cut into fillets

☐Fresh basil for garnish

☐Sea salt and pepper to taste

☐1 tablespoon olive oil (as a substitute for clarified butter)

☐Juice of one lemon, about 3 tablespoons

☐2 cloves garlic, minced

☐12 ounces spelt fettuccini, cooked (choose a lower sodium option)

☐20 spinach leaves

INSTRUCTIONS:

a)Preheat the oven to 375°F (190°C).

b)Season the salmon fillets with sea salt and pepper. Place them on a baking sheet lined with parchment paper.

c)Bake for about 15-20 minutes or until the salmon is cooked through. Flake it into bite-sized pieces.

d)Heat olive oil in a pan over medium heat. Add minced garlic and sauté for 1-2 minutes until fragrant.

e)Add the flaked salmon to the pan with garlic, and squeeze the lemon juice over the mixture. Stir gently to combine. In the pan with salmon, add the cooked spelt fettuccini and spinach leaves.

f)Toss until the spinach wilts and the ingredients are well combined. Garnish with fresh basil.

NUTRITION PER SERVING:

Calories: 350 | Protein: 20g | Fat: 10g | Carbohydrates: 40g | Fiber: 5g | Sodium: 150mg (adjusted for lower-sodium options) | Potassium: 300mg | Phosphorous: 150mg

BBQ CHICKEN QUINOA BOWL

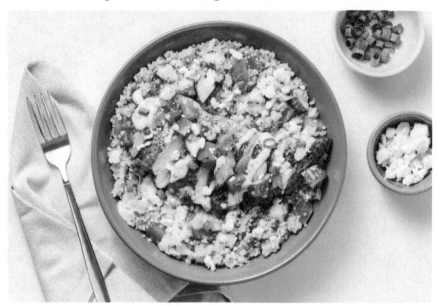

Makes: 1 serving

INGREDIENTS:

☐ ½ cup quinoa, rinsed

☐ 1 cup low-sodium chicken broth

☐ 1 boneless, skinless chicken breast (about 6 ounces)

☐ 2 tablespoons low-sodium barbecue sauce

☐ ½ cup low-potassium black beans, drained and rinsed

☐ ½ cup low-potassium corn kernels (fresh or frozen)

☐ ¼ cup red onion, finely chopped

☐ ¼ cup bell peppers, diced

☐ 1 tablespoon olive oil

☐ Salt and pepper to taste

☐ Fresh cilantro, chopped, for garnish (optional)

INSTRUCTIONS:

a)In a saucepan, combine quinoa and low-sodium chicken broth. Simmer for 15 minutes until quinoa is cooked and broth is absorbed. Season chicken breast with a small amount of salt and pepper.

b)Grill until fully cooked, brushing with a bit of low-sodium barbecue sauce in the last few minutes.

c)In a separate pan, heat olive oil over medium heat. Sauté red onion and bell peppers until softened.

d)Stir in black beans and corn, cooking until heated through. Place cooked quinoa in a bowl, and top with barbecue chicken, and black bean and corn mixture. Garnish with fresh cilantro if desired.

NUTRITION PER SERVING:

Calories: 400| Protein: 30g| Fat: 10g| Carbohydrates: 50g| Fiber: 7g| Sodium: 200mg| Potassium: 400mg| Phosphorus: 200mg

CHAPTER 4: SIDES AND SALADS

Welcome to Chapter 4 where we explore an enticing array of Sides and Salads that not only elevate your dining experience but also contribute to the well-being of your kidneys. Each recipe in this chapter is thoughtfully crafted to bring a burst of flavor and nutritional goodness to your table. From the satisfying crunch of Roasted Brussels with Turkey Bacon to the refreshing medley of Cucumber and Tomato Greek Salad, these sides and salads are a testament to the belief that maintaining renal health can be a vibrant and delicious endeavor. Indulge in the vibrant colors and textures of Turmeric Roasted Cauliflower, Beetroot and Feta Salad, and Kale and Berry Salad with Almonds, as you discover that nourishing your kidneys is a feast for the senses. Whether you're savoring the creamy goodness of Roasted Garlic Mashed Sweet Potatoes or delighting in the crispness of Snow Peas, Pine Nuts, and Asparagus Salad, each dish is a flavorful contribution to your commitment to renal well-being. So, join us in this exploration of sides and salads, where every bite is a celebration of taste and a step towards nurturing your kidneys.

ROASTED BRUSSELS WITH TURKEY BACON

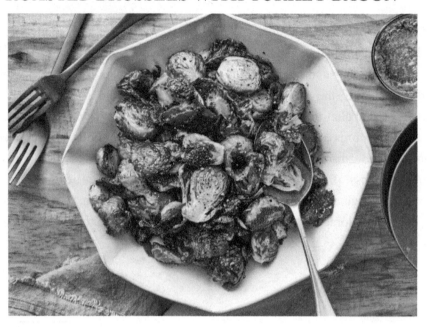

Makes: 4

INGREDIENTS:

☐1 pound whole Brussels sprouts

☐4 slices turkey bacon, cut into ½-inch pieces

☐½ teaspoon salt

☐¼ teaspoon freshly ground black pepper

☐2 tablespoons extra-virgin olive oil

☐1 tablespoon pure maple syrup (optional, and in moderation)

INSTRUCTIONS:

a)Preheat the oven to 400 degrees F (200 degrees C). Line a rimmed baking sheet with aluminum foil.

b)Trim ends off Brussels sprouts and cut any large ones in half. Transfer to a large bowl.

c)In a skillet over medium heat, cook the turkey bacon until it's slightly crispy. This might take a bit longer than regular bacon. Add the cooked turkey bacon, salt, and pepper to the Brussels sprouts. Drizzle olive oil over the top and toss until the sprouts are well coated. Transfer to the prepared baking sheet and spread in a single layer. Roast in the preheated oven for approximately 20 to 30 minutes, stirring halfway through.

d)If using, drizzle maple syrup over the Brussels sprouts during the last 5 minutes of roasting.

NUTRITION PER SERVING:

Calories: 120 | Protein: 5g | Fat: 7g | Carbohydrates: 10g | Fiber: 4g | Sodium: 300mg (adjusted for low-sodium preferences) | Potassium: 350mg | Phosphorus: 100mg

SPINACH, ARUGULA, AND AVOCADO SALAD

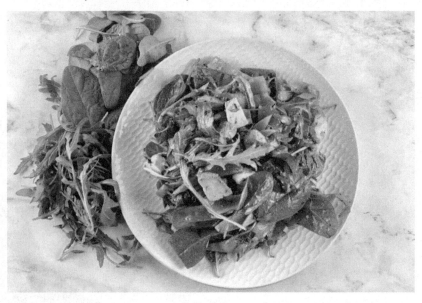

Makes: 4

INGREDIENTS:

☐3 ounces of baby arugula

☐2 ounces baby spinach

☐1 to 2 vine-ripe tomatoes, cut into wedges

☐½ English cucumber (or 1 slicing cucumber, peeled), halved lengthwise, then sliced

☐1 shallot, sliced

☐1 avocado, pitted and sliced

☐Renal-Friendly Vinaigrette

INSTRUCTIONS:

a)In a large mixing bowl, add the arugula, spinach, tomatoes, cucumbers, shallots, and sliced avocado.

b)Pour the renal-friendly vinaigrette over the salad ingredients.

c)Toss the salad gently to combine and coat evenly with the vinaigrette.

d)Taste and adjust seasoning if necessary.

e)Transfer the salad to a serving platter. Serve immediately.

NUTRITION PER SERVING:

Calories: 160 | Protein: 4g | Fat: 12g | Carbohydrates: 14g | Fiber: 5g | Sodium: 60mg (adjusted for low-sodium preferences) | Potassium: 350mg | Phosphorous: 70mg

CABBAGE AND CARROT COLESLAW

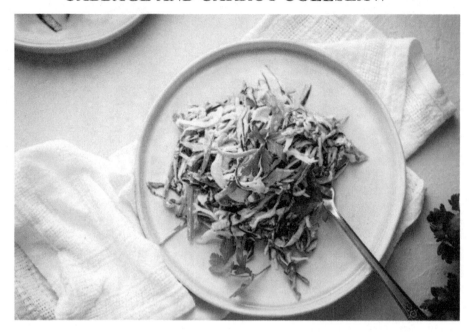

Makes: 2

INGREDIENTS:

☐ ½ shredded red cabbage

☐ ½ shredded green cabbage

☐ 1 carrot, sliced thin

☐ 1 courgette, sliced thin

☐ Handful of parsley

☐ ½ lime

☐ 1 chili

☐ 2 tablespoons of avocado oil

☐ Himalayan salt

INSTRUCTIONS:

a) Simply mix all the ingredients together in a mixing bowl, ensuring they are well combined.

b) Once everything is ready, it's time to sit back, relax, and Enjoy!

NUTRITION PER SERVING:

94 Calories: | Protein: 2 grams | Fat: 5 grams | Carbohydrates: 12 grams | Fiber: 3 grams | Sodium: 200mg | Potassium: 300mg | Phosphorus: 50mg

TURMERIC ROASTED CAULIFLOWER

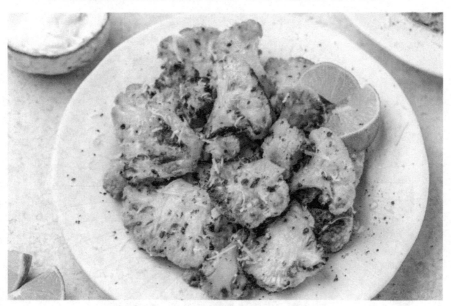

Makes: 5 Servings

INGREDIENTS:

☐ 8 cups cauliflower florets

☐ 3 tablespoons olive oil (extra-virgin)

☐ ½ teaspoon cumin powder

☐ ½ teaspoon of salt

☐ 2 teaspoons turmeric powder

☐ 2 teaspoons lemon juice

☐ ½ teaspoon black pepper

☐ 2 large garlic cloves, crushed

INSTRUCTIONS:

a) Preheat your oven to 425 °F.

b) In a bowl, combine oil, turmeric, cumin, salt, pepper, and garlic, and whisk them together.

c) Place the cauliflower on a rimmed baking sheet and coat it with the mixture.

d) Roast the cauliflower in the oven until it turns golden brown and becomes tender.

e) Once it's done, drizzle some lemon juice over the roasted cauliflower.

NUTRITION PER SERVING:

124 Calories: | Protein 3.5g | Carbohydrates 9.6 g | Dietary Fiber 3.7g | Sugar 3.3g | Fat 8.9g | Saturated Fat 1.4g | Sodium: 200mg | Potassium: 400mg | Phosphorus: 100mg

BEETROOT AND FETA SALAD

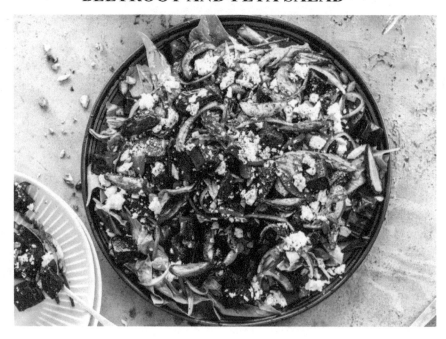

Makes: 4

INGREDIENTS:

☐3 tablespoons red wine vinegar, 1 teaspoon sugar, and ½ sliced red onion

☐3 large or 4 medium beetroot, peeled, cut into 1-1.5-inch cubes

☐Olive oil for cooking

☐½ cup chopped raw almonds

☐3 cloves garlic, chopped

☐4 ounces baby spinach and/or baby beetroot leaves

☐4-5 Medjool dates or 6-8 regular dried dates, chopped

☐2.5-3.5 ounces crumbled low-phosphorus feta

☐Extra virgin olive oil for dressing salad

INSTRUCTIONS:

a)Preheat the oven to 400°F. Line an oven tray with baking paper. On the lined tray, toss beetroot with a drizzle of olive oil and season with salt and pepper. Roast for 25-30 minutes or until tender.

b)In a bowl, mix red wine vinegar, sugar, and sliced red onion. Refrigerate for about 20 minutes.

c)Heat a drizzle of olive oil in a frying pan. Cook almonds and garlic for about 2 minutes until golden.

d)Drain the red onion and toss the vinegar with salad leaves, roasted beetroot, garlic almonds, dates, and crumbled feta. Dress with extra virgin olive oil and some reserved vinegar.

NUTRITION PER SERVING:

Calories: 250 | Protein: 6g | Fat: 12g | Carbohydrates: 30g | Fiber: 6g | Sodium: 150mg (adjusted for lower-sodium options) | Potassium: 300mg | Phosphorus: 120mg

ARUGULA AND PEAR SALAD WITH WALNUTS

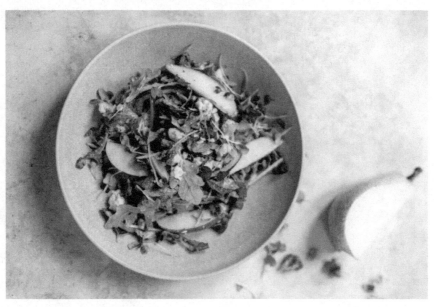

Makes: 8 Servings

INGREDIENTS:

☐4 cups arugula, trimmed, washed, and dried

☐2 firm red Bartlett pears, cut into 16 wedges

☐½ cup walnuts, chopped and toasted

☐5 cups butter-head lettuce

☐Your favorite dressing

INSTRUCTIONS:

a)Combine the lettuce, arugula, and dressing in a mixing bowl.

b)Sprinkle walnuts over the salad and serve it.

NUTRITION PER SERVING:

Calories: 125 | Total Fat: 8 g | Saturated Fat: 1 g | Sodium: 104 Mg | Total Carbohydrates: 10 g (Fiber: 3 g, Sugar: 5 g) | Protein: 2 g | Potassium: 250mg | Phosphorus: 80mg

SNOW PEAS, PINE NUTS, AND ASPARAGUS SALAD

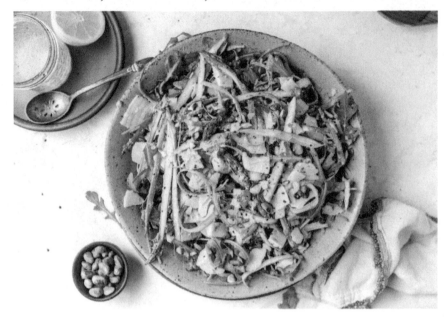

Makes: 2

INGREDIENTS:

☐ ½ cup snow peas, ends trimmed

☐ ½ cup asparagus, cut into bite-sized pieces

☐ ¼ cup pine nuts, toasted

☐ 1 tablespoon olive oil

☐ 1 tablespoon lemon juice

☐ 1 teaspoon Dijon mustard

☐ Salt and pepper to taste

☐ Fresh mint leaves for garnish (optional)

INSTRUCTIONS:

a) In a pot of boiling water, blanch snow peas and asparagus for about 2-3 minutes or until they are bright green and crisp-tender. Immediately transfer them to an ice bath to stop the cooking process. Drain and pat dry.

b) In a dry skillet, toast pine nuts over medium heat until golden brown. Be careful not to burn them.

c) In a bowl, whisk together olive oil, lemon juice, Dijon mustard, salt, and pepper to create the dressing.

d) Combine blanched snow peas, asparagus, and toasted pine nuts in a serving bowl.

e) Pour the dressing over the salad and toss to coat. Garnish with fresh mint leaves if desired.

NUTRITION PER SERVING:

Calories: 150 | Protein: 6 grams | Fat: 10 grams | Carbohydrates: 12 grams | Fiber: 5 grams | Sodium: 150mg | Potassium: 300mg | Phosphorus: 100mg

VEGGIE RATATOUILLE

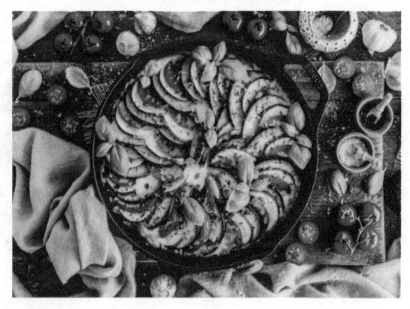

Makes: 4 Servings

INGREDIENTS:

☐1 tablespoon olive oil plus more for drizzling

☐1 onion, chopped

☐3 garlic cloves, minced

☐17.6 ounces strained tomatoes or passata

☐1 tablespoon tomato paste

☐1 tablespoon dried Italian herbs (e.g., basil, oregano, thyme)

☐1 zucchini, diced

☐1 small eggplant, diced

☐3 tomatoes, diced

INSTRUCTIONS:

a)In a large pot, heat 1-2 tablespoons of olive oil. Sauté chopped onion and minced garlic until soft.

b)Add strained tomatoes or low-potassium passata, and low-potassium tomato paste. Stir well.

c)Sprinkle dried Italian herbs, and stir to incorporate. Add diced zucchini, eggplant, and tomatoes. Stir gently to combine. Cover and simmer over low-medium heat for 20-25 minutes, or until vegetables are tender.

d)Drizzle with more olive oil, and garnish with fresh basil if desired.

NUTRITION PER SERVING:

Calories: 200 | Protein: 5g | Fat: 10g | Carbohydrates: 25g | Fiber: 8g | Sodium: 200mg (adjusted for low-sodium preferences) | Potassium: 500mg | Phosphorus: 80mg

KALE AND BERRY SALAD WITH ALMONDS

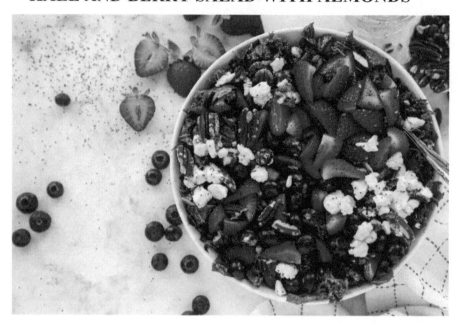

Makes: 4

INGREDIENTS:

6 cups fresh kale, stems removed, chopped

1 cup sliced strawberries, ½ cup blueberries, and ½ cup raspberries

½ cup almonds, chopped

¼ cup crumbled low-phosphorus feta cheese (optional)

FOR RENAL-FRIENDLY DRESSING:

3 tablespoons extra virgin olive oil

2 tablespoons balsamic vinegar (low sodium)

1 tablespoon honey

1 teaspoon Dijon mustard

Salt and pepper to taste

INSTRUCTIONS:

a)In a large mixing bowl, combine the chopped kale, strawberries, blueberries, raspberries, and almonds.

b)In a separate small bowl, whisk together the olive oil, balsamic vinegar, honey, Dijon mustard, salt, and pepper to create the dressing. Pour the dressing over the salad and toss gently to coat the ingredients evenly.

c)If desired, sprinkle crumbled feta cheese over the salad before serving.

NUTRITION PER SERVING:

Calories: 250 | Protein: 8g | Fat: 18g | Carbohydrates: 20g | Fiber: 5g | Sodium: 100mg (adjusted for low-sodium preferences) | Potassium: 400mg | Phosphorus: 120mg

ROASTED GARLIC MASHED SWEET POTATOES

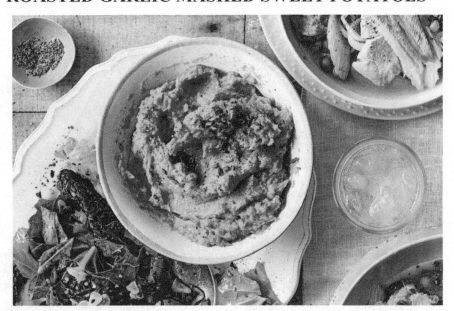

Makes: 4 servings

INGREDIENTS:

☐2 large sweet potatoes, peeled and cubed

☐2 cloves garlic, minced

☐2 tablespoons olive oil

☐¼ cup low-sodium vegetable broth

☐Salt and pepper to taste

☐Chopped chives for garnish (optional)

INSTRUCTIONS:

a)Preheat the oven to 400°F (200°C).

b)Toss sweet potato cubes and minced garlic with olive oil, salt, and pepper in a bowl.

c)Spread the sweet potatoes on a baking sheet and roast for 25-30 minutes or until tender, stirring halfway through. Transfer roasted sweet potatoes to a bowl and mash with a fork or potato masher.

d)Gradually add vegetable broth while continuing to mash until you achieve your desired consistency.

e)Season with additional salt and pepper if needed.

f)Garnish with chopped chives if desired.

NUTRITION PER SERVING:

Calories: 180| Protein: 2g| Fat: 7g| Carbohydrates: 30g| Fiber: 4g| Sodium: 70mg| Potassium: 400mg| Phosphorous: 80mg

ROASTED BRUSSELS SPROUTS AND BUTTERNUT SQUASH

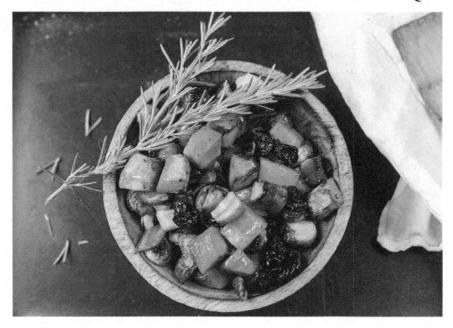

Makes: 4

INGREDIENTS:

□1 pound Brussels sprouts, trimmed and halved

□1 small butternut squash, peeled, seeded, and cut into cubes

□2 tablespoons olive oil

□2 cloves garlic, minced

□1 teaspoon dried thyme

□Salt and pepper to taste

□¼ cup chopped pecans (optional)

INSTRUCTIONS:

a)Preheat the oven to 400°F (200°C).

b)In a large mixing bowl, combine the halved Brussels sprouts and cubed butternut squash.

c)In a small bowl, mix together the olive oil, minced garlic, dried thyme, salt, and pepper.

d)Drizzle the olive oil mixture over the vegetables and toss until well coated.

e)Spread the vegetables in a single layer on a baking sheet.

f)Roast in the preheated oven for about 25-30 minutes or until the Brussels sprouts are golden brown and the butternut squash is tender. Stir halfway through the roasting time for even cooking.

g)If using, sprinkle chopped pecans over the vegetables during the last 5 minutes of roasting.

NUTRITION PER SERVING:

Calories: 150 | Protein: 3g | Fat: 8g | Carbohydrates: 20g | Fiber: 6g | Sodium: 30mg | Potassium: 500mg | Phosphorus: 70mg

CUCUMBER AND TOMATO GREEK SALAD

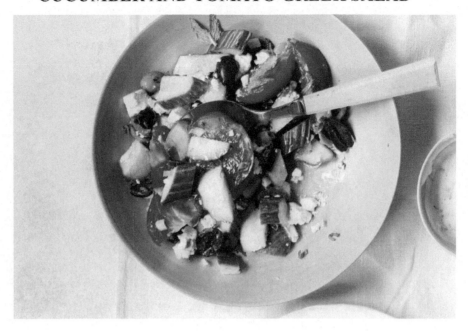

Makes: 4

INGREDIENTS:

☐2 large cucumbers, diced

☐4 medium tomatoes, diced

☐½ red onion, thinly sliced

☐½ cup Kalamata olives, pitted and sliced

☐½ cup crumbled feta cheese (low-phosphorus option)

☐¼ cup extra virgin olive oil

☐2 tablespoons red wine vinegar (low sodium)

☐1 teaspoon dried oregano

☐Salt and pepper to taste

☐Fresh parsley for garnish (optional)

INSTRUCTIONS:

a)In a large mixing bowl, combine diced cucumbers, diced tomatoes, sliced red onion, Kalamata olives, and crumbled feta cheese.

b)In a small bowl, whisk together the extra virgin olive oil, red wine vinegar, dried oregano, salt, and pepper to create the dressing. Pour the dressing over the salad and toss gently to coat the ingredients evenly.

c)Garnish with fresh parsley if desired. Serve immediately and enjoy.

NUTRITION PER SERVING:

Calories: 200 | Protein: 5g | Fat: 15g | Carbohydrates: 15g | Fiber: 4g | Sodium: 300mg (adjusted for low-sodium preferences) | Potassium: 500mg | Phosphorus: 120mg

SPINACH AND STRAWBERRY SALAD

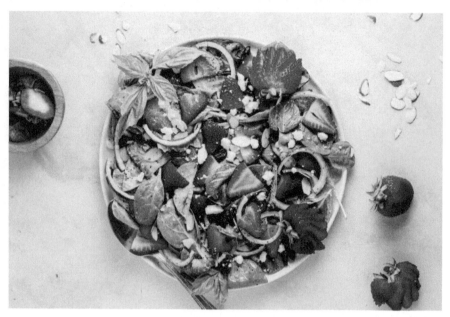

Makes: 4

INGREDIENTS:

☐6 cups fresh spinach leaves, washed and stems removed

☐2 cups strawberries, hulled and sliced

☐½ cup red onion, thinly sliced

☐¼ cup chopped walnuts or almonds (optional)

☐¼ cup crumbled feta cheese (low-phosphorus option)

FOR RENAL-FRIENDLY DRESSING:

☐3 tablespoons extra virgin olive oil

☐2 tablespoons balsamic vinegar (low sodium)

☐1 tablespoon honey

☐1 teaspoon Dijon mustard

☐Salt and pepper to taste

INSTRUCTIONS:

a)Mix fresh spinach, sliced strawberries, red onion, and optional nuts in a bowl.

b)Whisk together olive oil, balsamic vinegar, honey, Dijon mustard, salt, and pepper for the dressing.

c)Pour the dressing over the salad, and toss gently to coat evenly. Sprinkle feta cheese before serving.

NUTRITION PER SERVING:

Calories: 200 | Protein: 4g | Fat: 15g | Carbohydrates: 15g | Fiber: 4g | Sodium: 150mg (adjusted for low-sodium preferences) | Potassium: 500mg | Phosphorus: 120mg

AVOCADO AND TOMATO CAPRESE SALAD

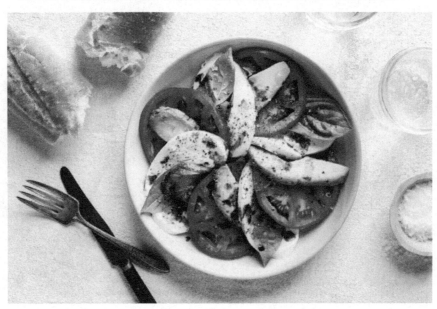

Makes: 4

INGREDIENTS:

☐2 large tomatoes, sliced

☐2 ripe avocados, sliced

☐1 cup fresh mozzarella, sliced

☐Fresh basil leaves, for garnish

☐Balsamic glaze (low-sodium) for drizzling

☐Extra virgin olive oil for drizzling

☐Salt and pepper to taste

INSTRUCTIONS:

a)On a serving platter, arrange the tomato slices, avocado slices, and fresh mozzarella slices in an alternating pattern. Tuck fresh basil leaves between the slices.

b)Drizzle balsamic glaze and extra virgin olive oil over the salad.

c)Sprinkle with a pinch of salt and pepper to taste.

d)Garnish with additional fresh basil leaves.

e)Serve immediately and enjoy your Renal-Friendly Avocado and Tomato Caprese Salad!

NUTRITION PER SERVING:

Calories: 250 | Protein: 8g | Fat: 20g | Carbohydrates: 10g | Fiber: 6g | Sodium: 150mg (adjusted for low-sodium preferences) | Potassium: 700mg | Phosphorus: 120mg

GARLIC AND HERB MASHED CAULIFLOWER

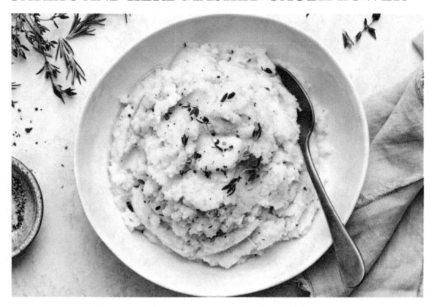

Makes: 4

INGREDIENTS:

☐1 head of cauliflower florets, rinsed

☐1 tablespoon extra-virgin olive oil

☐2 garlic cloves, minced

☐1 to 2 teaspoons finely chopped herbs (such as thyme, rosemary, sage, parsley, chives, etc.)

☐Salt and pepper to taste

INSTRUCTIONS:

a)Heat 1 inch of water in a pot on medium heat and bring to a boil. Place a steamer insert in the pot and add the cauliflower florets. Steam for 6 to 8 minutes.

b)While the cauliflower is steaming, heat the olive oil in a small pan on medium heat. Add the minced garlic and cook for 30 seconds, then remove from the heat.

c)Remove the steamed cauliflower from the pot, drain the water, and add the cauliflower back in. Then, add the olive oil, garlic, chopped renal-friendly herbs, and any optional ingredients.

d)Use a potato masher or stick blender to mash the cauliflower.

e)Season with salt and pepper, garnish with fresh renal-friendly herbs, and serve immediately.

NUTRITION PER SERVING:

Calories: 60 | Protein: 2g | Fat: 3g | Carbohydrates: 8g | Fiber: 4g | Sodium: 30mg | Potassium: 300mg | Phosphorus: 50mg

ARUGULA AND POMEGRANATE SALAD

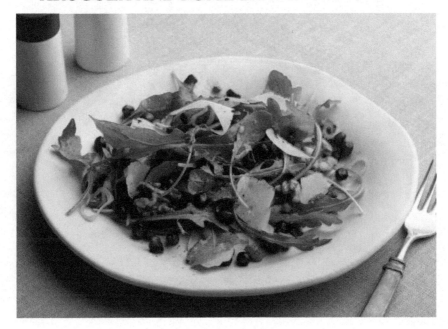

Makes: 4

INGREDIENTS:
FOR THE SALAD:

☐6 cups arugula, washed and dried

☐1 cup pomegranate seeds

☐½ cup crumbled low-phosphorus feta cheese (optional)

☐¼ cup chopped walnuts or almonds (optional)

FOR THE DRESSING:

☐3 tablespoons extra virgin olive oil

☐2 tablespoons balsamic vinegar (low sodium)

☐1 tablespoon honey

☐1 teaspoon Dijon mustard

☐Salt and pepper to taste

INSTRUCTIONS:

a)Mix arugula, pomegranate seeds, and optional feta cheese and nuts in a large bowl.

b)Whisk together olive oil, balsamic vinegar, honey, Dijon mustard, salt, and pepper for the dressing.

c)Pour dressing over the salad, and toss gently to coat evenly.

NUTRITION PER SERVING:

Calories: 200 | Protein: 4g | Fat: 15g | Carbohydrates: 15g | Fiber: 4g | Sodium: 150mg (adjusted for low-sodium preferences) | Potassium: 400mg | Phosphorus: 120mg

ALMOND BALSAMIC BEANS

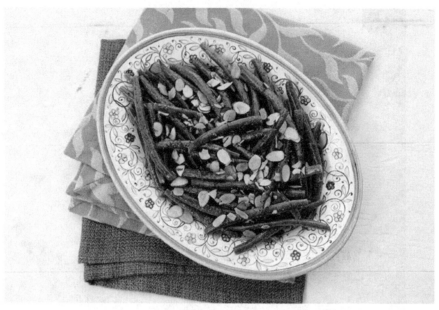

Makes: 4 Servings

INGREDIENTS:
- 2 tablespoons ground almonds
- 1 pound green beans
- 1 tablespoon olive oil
- 1½ tablespoons balsamic vinegar

INSTRUCTIONS:
a)Cook the green beans by steaming them along with a mixture of olive oil and balsamic vinegar.

b)Just before serving, incorporate the almonds into the dish.

NUTRITION PER SERVING:
Calories: 150 | Protein: 6 grams | Fat: 7 grams | Carbohydrates: 16 grams | Fiber: 5 grams | Sodium: 200mg | Potassium: 250mg | Phosphorus: 120mg

KALE SLAW AND CREAMY DRESSING

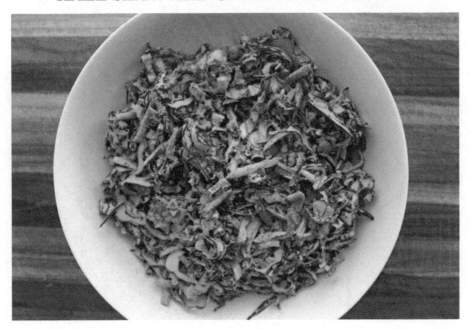

Makes: 4

INGREDIENTS:
FOR THE SLAW:
☐4 cups kale, stems removed, finely chopped

☐2 cups cabbage, shredded

☐1 carrot, grated

☐¼ cup red onion, thinly sliced

FOR THE CREAMY DRESSING:
☐½ cup plain Greek yogurt (low-phosphorus option)

☐2 tablespoons mayonnaise (low-phosphorus option)

☐2 tablespoons apple cider vinegar

☐1 tablespoon honey

☐1 teaspoon Dijon mustard

☐Salt and pepper to taste

INSTRUCTIONS:
a)Mix kale, shredded cabbage, grated carrot, and sliced red onion in a bowl.

b)Whisk together Greek yogurt, mayonnaise, apple cider vinegar, honey, Dijon mustard, salt, and pepper.

c)Pour dressing over slaw ingredients. Toss gently to coat evenly. Serve immediately or refrigerate.

NUTRITION PER SERVING:
Calories: 150 | Protein: 5g | Fat: 8g | Carbohydrates: 15g | Fiber: 5g | Sodium: 150mg (adjusted for low-sodium preferences) | Potassium: 400mg | Phosphorus: 120mg

STEAMED ASPARAGUS WITH CAPERS AND LEMON

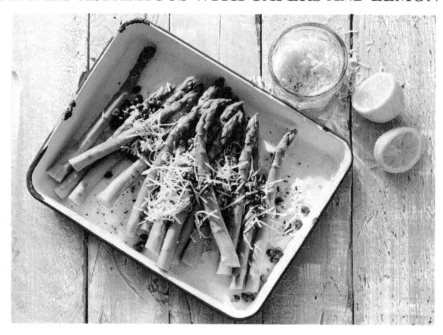

Makes: 4

INGREDIENTS:

☐1 bunch of asparagus, woody ends trimmed

☐1 tablespoon olive oil

☐2 tablespoons capers, drained

☐Zest of 1 lemon

☐Juice of 1 lemon

☐Salt and pepper to taste

INSTRUCTIONS:

a)Trim the woody ends from the asparagus spears.

b)Steam the asparagus until tender-crisp, about 4-5 minutes.

c)In a small pan, heat olive oil over low heat. Add capers and sauté for 1-2 minutes until they start to crisp.

d)Remove the pan from heat and add lemon zest and lemon juice to the capers. Stir well.

e)Arrange the steamed asparagus on a serving plate.

f)Pour the caper and lemon mixture over the asparagus.

g)Season with salt and pepper to taste.

h)Serve warm and enjoy.

NUTRITION PER SERVING:

Calories: 50 | Protein: 2g | Fat: 3g | Carbohydrates: 5g | Fiber: 2g | Sodium: 150mg (adjusted for low-sodium preferences) | Potassium: 200mg | Phosphorus: 40mg

MIXED GREEN SPRING SALAD

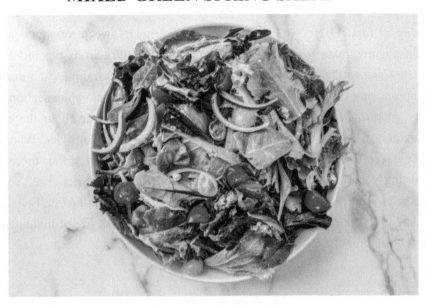

Makes: 1 serving

INGREDIENTS:

2 cups mixed renal-friendly salad greens (e.g., spinach, arugula, romaine)

½ cucumber, thinly sliced

½ red bell pepper, thinly sliced

1 tablespoon Kalamata olives, sliced

1 tablespoon cherry tomatoes, halved

1 tablespoon feta cheese, crumbled (low-phosphorus option)

1 tablespoon red onion, thinly sliced

2 tablespoons extra virgin olive oil

1 tablespoon balsamic vinegar (low sodium)

1 teaspoon Dijon mustard

Salt and pepper to taste

INSTRUCTIONS:

a)In a large renal-friendly salad bowl, combine mixed salad greens, sliced cucumber, sliced red bell pepper, Kalamata olives, cherry tomatoes, crumbled low-phosphorus feta cheese, and thinly sliced red onion.

b)In a small bowl, whisk together extra virgin olive oil, balsamic vinegar, Dijon mustard, salt, and pepper to create the dressing. Drizzle the dressing over the salad and toss gently to coat all ingredients.

NUTRITION PER SERVING:

Calories: 250 | Protein: 5g | Fat: 20g | Carbohydrates: 15g | Fiber: 5g | Potassium: 400mg | Phosphorus: 100mg

CHAPTER 5: DESSERTS

Welcome to the sweet finale. Here, we present a delightful array of sweet treats meticulously crafted to satisfy your cravings while aligning with your commitment to renal health. From the indulgent richness of Low-Phosphorus Chocolate Cake to the refreshing allure of Assorted Berry Granita, each dessert is a celebration of flavors without compromising on kidney-friendly choices. Savor the sweet sophistication of Lemon Poppy Seed Cake or the creamy goodness of Avocado Pudding with Nuts. Treat yourself to the comforting nostalgia of Oatmeal Raisin Cookies or the tropical delight of Pineapple Coconut Chia Popsicles. Whether you're relishing the elegance of Mini Pavlovas or the guilt-free pleasure of No-Bake Blueberry Pie, these desserts invite you to discover that supporting your kidneys can be a delightful and flavorful experience. So, join us in this sweet journey through Desserts, where each recipe, from Vanilla Poached Pears to Frozen Banana Bites, is a delectable reminder that nourishing your kidneys doesn't mean compromising on the joy of indulgence. Let every bite be a celebration of both taste and renal well-being.

LOW-PHOSPHORUS CHOCOLATE CAKE

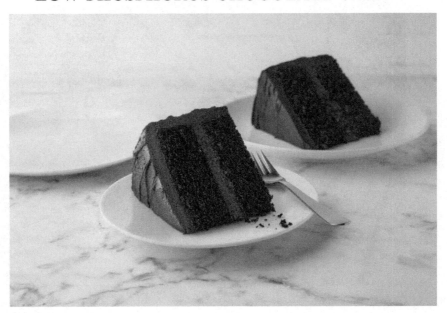

Makes: One 8-inch cake

INGREDIENTS:

☐ 1 cup almond flour

☐ ½ cup cocoa powder (unsweetened)

☐ ½ cup erythritol (or sweetener of your choice)

☐ 1 teaspoon baking powder

☐ ¼ teaspoon salt

☐ ½ cup unsweetened applesauce

☐ 3 large eggs

☐ ¼ cup coconut oil, melted

☐ 1 teaspoon vanilla extract

INSTRUCTIONS:

a) Preheat your oven to 350°F (175°C) and grease a cake pan.

b) In a large bowl, mix almond flour, cocoa powder, erythritol, baking powder, and salt.

c) Add applesauce, eggs, melted coconut oil, and vanilla extract to the dry ingredients. Mix until well combined. Pour the batter into the prepared cake pan and spread it evenly.

d) Bake for 25-30 minutes or until a toothpick inserted into the center comes out clean.

e) Allow the cake to cool completely before frosting.

NUTRITION PER SERVING:

Calories: 150 | Protein: 5g | Fat: 12g | Carbohydrates: 8g | Fiber: 3g | Sodium: 80mg | Potassium: 120mg | Phosphorous: 80mg

LEMON POPPY SEED CAKE

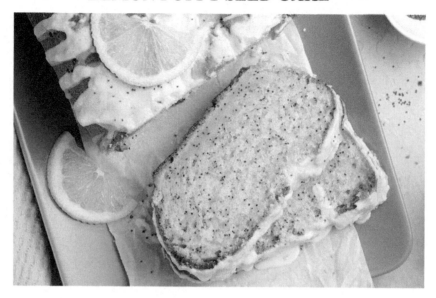

Makes: 1 loaf

INGREDIENTS:

☐1 ½ cups all-purpose flour

☐½ cup kidney-friendly sweetener (e.g., erythritol or stevia)

☐1 tablespoon poppy seeds

☐½ teaspoon baking powder

☐¼ teaspoon baking soda

☐¼ teaspoon low sodium salt

☐½ cup unsalted butter, softened

☐2 large eggs

☐½ cup low-phosphorus milk (e.g., almond milk or rice milk)

☐1 tablespoon fresh lemon juice

☐Zest of 1 lemon

INSTRUCTIONS:

a)Preheat oven to 350°F (175°C). Grease and flour loaf pan.

b)Whisk together flour, kidney-friendly sweetener, poppy seeds, baking powder, baking soda, and salt. Set aside. Cream softened butter and kidney-friendly sweetener in a large bowl until fluffy.

c)Add eggs one at a time, beating well after each addition. Gradually add dry ingredients to wet ingredients. Stir in lemon juice and lemon zest. Pour batter into the prepared loaf pan, and smooth the top.

d)Bake for 45-50 minutes. Cool in pan for 10 minutes, then transfer to a wire rack to cool completely.

NUTRITION PER SERVING:

Calories: 130 | Protein: 2g | Fat: 9g | Carbohydrates: 10g | Fiber: 1g | Sodium: 75mg | Potassium: 20mg | Phosphorous: 30mg

ASSORTED BERRY GRANITA

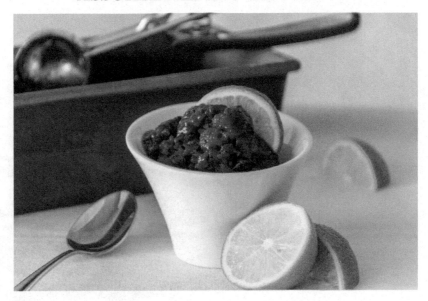

Makes: 4

INGREDIENTS:

☐ ½ cup fresh strawberries, peeled and sliced

☐ ½ cup of fresh raspberries

☐ ½ cup of fresh blueberries

☐ ½ cup fresh blackberries

☐ 1 tablespoon of maple syrup

☐ 1 tablespoon fresh lemon juice

☐ 1 cup ice cubes, crushed

INSTRUCTIONS:

a) Add berries, maple syrup, lemon juice, and ice cubes to a high-speed blender. Blend on high speed until the mixture becomes smooth.

b) Pour the blended berry mixture into an 8 x 8-inch baking dish, ensuring it is spread evenly. Place the dish in the freezer and let it freeze for a minimum of 30 minutes.

c) Remove the baking dish from the freezer and use a fork to thoroughly stir the granita until it is well mixed.

d) Place the dish back in the freezer and allow it to freeze for 2-3 hours, making sure to stir the mixture every 30 minutes.

NUTRITION PER SERVING:

Calories: 46 | Fat: 0.3g | Carbohydrates: 11g | Fiber: 2.8g | Sugars: 7.3g | Protein: 0.7g | Sodium: 0mg | Potassium: 100mg | Phosphorus: 15mg

DATE AND PUMPKIN ICE CREAM

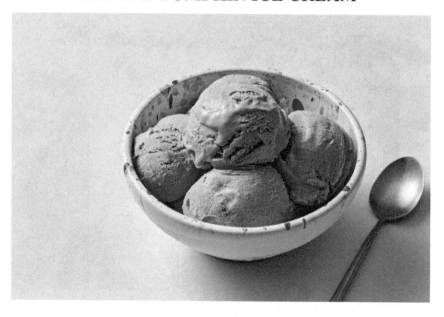

Makes: 6

INGREDIENTS:

☐15 ounces of home-made pumpkin purée

☐½ cup dates, pitted and chopped

☐2 cans (14 ounces) of unsweetened coconut milk

☐½ teaspoon organic vanilla extract

☐1½ teaspoons pumpkin pie spice

☐½ teaspoon ground cinnamon

INSTRUCTIONS:

a)Combine all the ingredients in a blender and blend until a smooth mixture is obtained.

b)Transfer the mixture to a container suitable for freezing and place it in the freezer for a maximum of 2 hours.

c)Remove the partially frozen mixture from the freezer and pour it into an ice cream maker. Follow the manufacturer's instructions to process the mixture.

d)Once the processing is complete, transfer the ice cream to a freezer-safe container and freeze it for an additional 2 hours before serving.

NUTRITION PER SERVING:

Calories: 100 | Protein: 2 grams | Fat: 3 grams | Carbohydrates: 18 grams | Fiber: 4 grams | Sodium: 30mg | Potassium: 200mg | Phosphorus: 70mg

AVOCADO PUDDING WITH NUTS

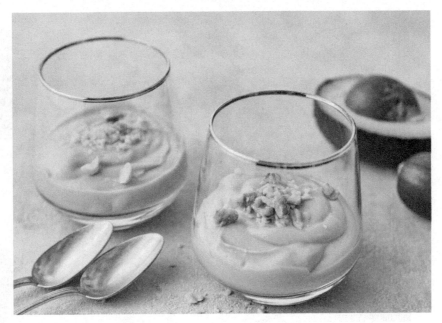

Makes: 3 Servings

INGREDIENTS:

☐2 ripe avocados

☐⅔ cup unsweetened almond milk (choose a low-phosphorus option)

☐3 tablespoons artificial sweetener e.g., Xylitol

☐1 teaspoon lemon juice

☐Pinch of salt (optional)

☐Nuts, to top (choose low-phosphorus options, like almonds or pistachios)

INSTRUCTIONS:

a)Place the avocados, almond milk, artificial sweetener, lemon juice, and salt (if using) in a blender and blend until well processed. Alternatively, you can use an immersion blender to cream all the ingredients together.

b)Chill the pudding in the refrigerator for about an hour.

c)Before serving, top the pudding with nuts of your choice.

d)Enjoy your Renal-Friendly Avocado Pudding!

NUTRITION PER SERVING:

Calories: 200 | Protein: 3g | Fat: 15g | Carbohydrates: 15g | Fiber: 7g | Sodium: 50mg | Potassium: 400mg | Phosphorus: 70mg

STRAWBERRY SOUFFLÉ

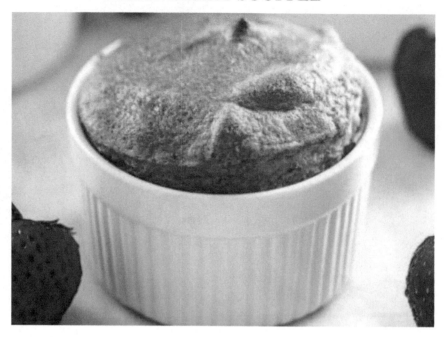

Makes: 6

INGREDIENTS:

☐18 ounces fresh strawberries, peeled and puréed

☐⅓ cup raw honey

☐5 organic egg whites

☐4 teaspoons fresh lemon juice

INSTRUCTIONS:

a)Start by preheating your oven to 350ºF (175ºC).

b)In a bowl, combine the strawberry purée, 3 tablespoons of honey, 2 egg whites, and lemon juice. Pulse the mixture until it becomes fluffy and light.

c)In a separate bowl, beat the remaining egg whites until they become fluffy.

d)Mix in the remaining honey with the beaten egg whites.

e)Gently stir the beaten egg whites into the strawberry mixture.

f)Evenly distribute the resulting mixture into 6 ramekins placed on a baking sheet.

g)Place the baking sheet with the ramekins in the oven and bake for approximately 10-12 minutes.

h)Once cooked, remove from the oven and serve immediately.

NUTRITION PER SERVING:

Calories: 180 | Fat: 0.3g | Carbohydrates: 22.3g | Fiber: 1.8g | Sugars: 19.9g | Protein: 3.7g | Sodium: 21.1mg | Potassium: 220 milligram | Phosphorus: 100mg

PUMPKIN PIE

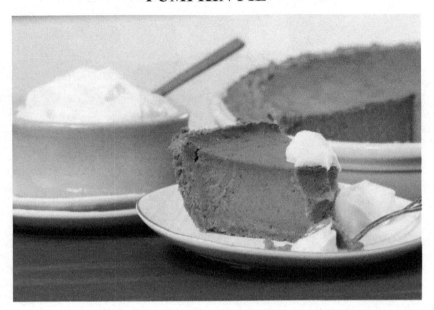

Makes: 8 Servings

INGREDIENTS:

☐1 pre-made or homemade low-sodium graham cracker crust

☐15 ounces canned pumpkin puree (unsweetened)

☐2 large eggs

☐1 cup low-phosphorus milk (e.g., almond milk)

☐½ cup kidney-friendly sweetener (e.g., sucralose)

☐1 teaspoon ground cinnamon

☐½ teaspoon ground ginger

☐¼ teaspoon ground nutmeg

☐¼ teaspoon salt

INSTRUCTIONS:

a)Preheat the oven to 425°F (220°C).

b)In a large bowl, whisk together pumpkin puree, eggs, low-phosphorus milk, kidney-friendly sweetener, cinnamon, ginger, nutmeg, and salt until well combined. Pour the pumpkin mixture into the graham cracker crust. Bake in the preheated oven for 15 minutes. Reduce the oven temperature to 350°F (175°C) and continue baking for an additional 35-40 minutes or until a knife inserted into the center comes out clean.

c)Allow the pumpkin pie to cool completely before refrigerating.

d)Refrigerate for at least 4 hours or overnight to allow the pie to set. Slice and serve chilled.

NUTRITION PER SERVING:

Calories: 180| Protein: 4g| Fat: 8g| Carbohydrates: 25g| Fiber: 3g| Sodium: 180mg| Potassium: 200mg| Phosphorous: 80mg

SPICY ZUCCHINI BROWNIES

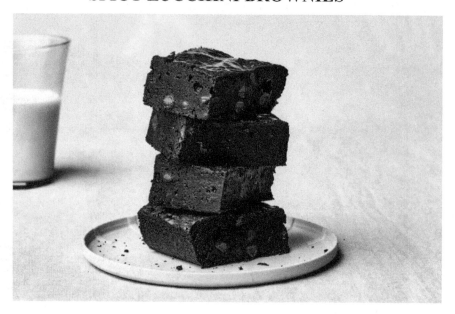

Makes: 20

INGREDIENTS:

☐ 1½ cups zucchini, grated

☐ 1 cup dark chocolate chips

☐ 1 egg

☐ 1 cup almond butter

☐ ⅓ cup raw honey

☐ 1 teaspoon baking powder

☐ 1 teaspoon ground cinnamon

☐ ½ teaspoon ground nutmeg

☐ 1 teaspoon vanilla extract

INSTRUCTIONS:

a)Start by preheating your oven to 350ºF (175ºC) and greasing a baking dish.

b)In a bowl, mix together all of the ingredients until well combined. Pour the resulting mixture into the prepared baking dish.

c)Place the baking dish in the preheated oven and bake for approximately 40 minutes, or until the dish is cooked through.

d)Once done, remove the dish from the oven and cut it into squares. Serve and enjoy.

NUTRITION PER SERVING:

Calories: 180 | Protein: 4 grams | Fat: 9 grams | Carbohydrates: 24 grams | Fiber: 3 grams | Sodium: 150mg | Potassium: 220mg | Phosphorus: 100mg

WHITE CHOCOLATE PUDDING WITH RASPBERRY SAUCE

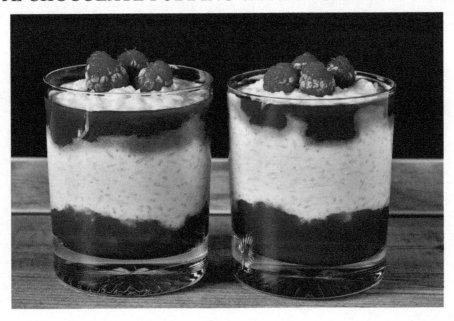

Makes: 4

INGREDIENTS:

☐1 cup white rice, rinsed and drained

☐4 cups unsweetened almond milk (choose a low-phosphorus option)

☐¼ cup artificial sweetener suitable for a renal diet (e.g., sucralose)

☐Zest of 1 lemon

☐¼ cup white chocolate chips (choose a low-phosphorus option)

☐1 teaspoon vanilla extract

☐Pinch of salt

☐½ cup unsweetened Raspberry Dessert Sauce

INSTRUCTIONS:

a)In a medium-sized pot, combine rinsed white rice, almond milk, artificial sweetener, lemon zest, and a pinch of salt.

b)Bring the mixture to a boil, then reduce the heat to low. Cover and simmer for 20-25 minutes, or until the rice is tender, stirring occasionally.

c)Stir in white chocolate chips and vanilla extract, and continue cooking for an additional 5 minutes until the pudding thickens. Remove from heat and let it cool. Drizzle each serving with raspberry sauce.

d)Optionally, garnish with additional lemon zest or fresh raspberries.

NUTRITION PER SERVING:

Calories: 200 | Protein: 4g | Fat: 6g | Carbohydrates: 30g | Fiber: 3g | Sodium: 80mg | Potassium: 150mg | Phosphorus: 70mg

PEACH SORBET

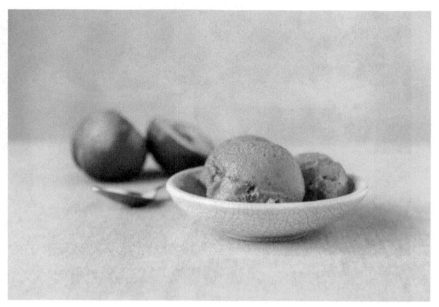

Makes: 2 Servings

INGREDIENTS:

☐4 ripe peaches, peeled and pitted

☐¼ cup water

☐2 tablespoons lemon juice

☐Kidney-friendly sweetener to taste (optional)

INSTRUCTIONS:

a)Start by dicing the peaches and placing them in a blender or food processor.

b)Combine water and lemon juice with the diced peaches in the blender.

c)Blend the ingredients until they form a smooth mixture.

d)Sample the mixture and add a suitable sweetener for those with kidney concerns, if desired.

e)Transfer the blended mixture to a shallow dish and place it in the freezer. Stir the mixture every hour for 3-4 hours until the sorbet reaches the desired consistency.

f)Present the sorbet in small bowls or glasses for serving.

NUTRITION PER SERVING:

Calories: 80 | Protein: 1g | Fat: 0g | Carbohydrates: 20g | Fiber: 2g | Sodium: 0mg | Potassium: 220mg | Phosphorus: 20mg

OATMEAL RAISIN COOKIES

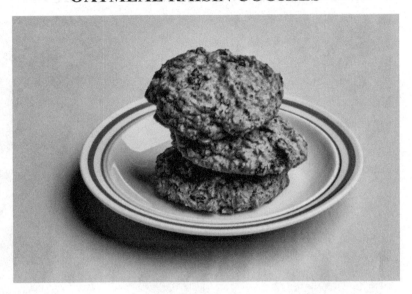

Makes: 2 Servings

INGREDIENTS:

☐ 1 cup rolled oats

☐ ½ cup all-purpose flour

☐ ½ teaspoon baking powder

☐ ¼ teaspoon salt

☐ ¼ cup unsalted butter, softened

☐ ½ cup kidney-friendly sweetener (e.g., erythritol)

☐ 1 large egg

☐ 1 teaspoon vanilla extract

☐ ½ cup raisins

INSTRUCTIONS:

a)Begin by preheating your oven to 350°F (175°C) and preparing a baking sheet with parchment paper.

b)In a bowl, combine oats, flour, baking powder, and salt, whisking them together.

c)In a separate bowl, cream together softened butter and sweetener until the mixture becomes fluffy.

d)Add the egg and vanilla extract to the creamy mixture, beating them in until well incorporated.

e)Gradually incorporate the dry ingredients into the wet ingredients, mixing until just combined.

f)Gently stir in the raisins. Using rounded tablespoons of dough, drop portions onto the lined baking sheet.

g)Bake the cookies for 10 to 12 minutes, or until you notice the edges turning a light golden color.

NUTRITION PER SERVING:

Calories: 130 | Protein: 2g | Fat: 5g | Carbohydrates: 20g | Potassium: 70mg | Phosphorus: 40mg

PINEAPPLE COCONUT CHIA POPSICLES

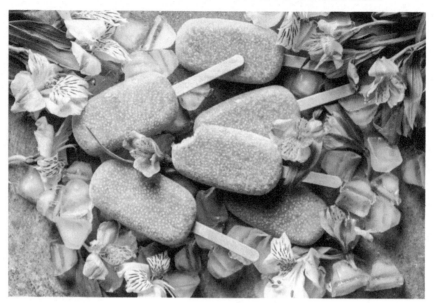

Makes: 2 Servings

INGREDIENTS:

- 1 cup unsweetened coconut milk
- 1 cup fresh pineapple chunks
- 2 tablespoons chia seeds
- 1 tablespoon kidney-friendly sweetener (e.g., erythritol) (optional)

INSTRUCTIONS:

a)Place coconut milk, pineapple chunks, and optionally a sweetener suitable for those with kidney concerns, into a blender.

b)Blend the ingredients until a smooth consistency is achieved.

c)Add chia seeds to the mixture and allow it to sit for 10 minutes to thicken.

d)Pour the thickened mixture into popsicle molds.

e)Place the molds in the freezer for a minimum of 4 hours, or until the popsicles are completely frozen.

f)Take the popsicles out of the molds and serve them.

NUTRITION PER SERVING:

Calories: 90 | Protein: 2 g | Fat: 5 g | Carbohydrates: 10 g | Fiber: 3 g | Sodium: 10 mg | Potassium: 150 mg | Phosphorous: 50 mg

MINI PAVLOVAS

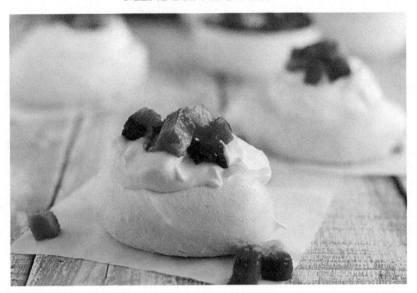

Makes: 12 mini pavlovas

INGREDIENTS:
FOR THE PAVLOVAS:
☐4 large egg whites, at room temperature

☐1 cup granulated sugar

☐1 teaspoon white vinegar

☐1 teaspoon cornstarch

☐½ teaspoon vanilla extract

FOR THE TOPPING:
☐1 cup whipped cream

☐Fresh berries (strawberries, blueberries, raspberries)

☐Mint leaves for garnish

☐Powdered sugar for dusting

INSTRUCTIONS:
a)Preheat oven to 275°F (135°C). Line the baking sheet with parchment paper.

b)Beat egg whites in a clean bowl until soft peaks form. Gradually add sugar, beating until stiff peaks form. Mix in vinegar, cornstarch, and vanilla; gently fold. Spoon meringue onto the sheet, forming nests with indentations. Bake for 60-70 mins until crisp and slightly pale.

c)Cool pavlovas in the turned-off oven to prevent cracking. Carefully remove cooled pavlovas from the parchment. Fill with whipped cream. Top with fresh berries. Garnish with mint leaves and powdered sugar.

NUTRITION PER SERVING:
Calories: 150 | Protein: 1g | Fat: 5g | Carbohydrates: 26g | Fiber: 1g | Sodium: 20mg | Potassium: 50mg | Phosphorous: 20mg

NO-BAKE BLUEBERRY PIE

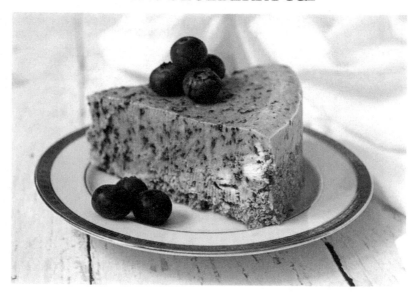

Makes: 1 pie

INGREDIENTS:

☐2 cups fresh blueberries

☐1 pre-made graham cracker crust (9 inches)

☐1 package (8 ounces) cream cheese, softened

☐½ cup powdered sugar

☐1 teaspoon vanilla extract

☐1 cup whipped topping (sugar-free)

☐Fresh mint leaves for garnish (optional)

INSTRUCTIONS:

a)In a medium-sized bowl, gently fold 1 cup of blueberries. Set aside the remaining blueberries for later.

b)In a separate mixing bowl, beat the cream cheese until smooth.

c)Add powdered sugar and vanilla extract to the cream cheese, continuing to beat until well combined.

d)Gently fold in the whipped topping until the mixture is smooth and creamy.

e)Carefully fold in the blueberry mixture until evenly distributed.

f)Spoon the blueberry mixture into the graham cracker crust, spreading it evenly.

g)Chill the pie in the refrigerator for at least 2 hours or until set.

h)Before serving, top the pie with the remaining fresh blueberries and garnish with mint leaves if desired.

NUTRITION PER SERVING:

Calories: 300 | Protein: 2g | Fat: 14g | Carbohydrates: 44g | Fiber: 2g | Sodium: 220mg | Potassium: 100mg | Phosphorous: 40mg

RASPBERRY CHEESECAKE MOUSSE

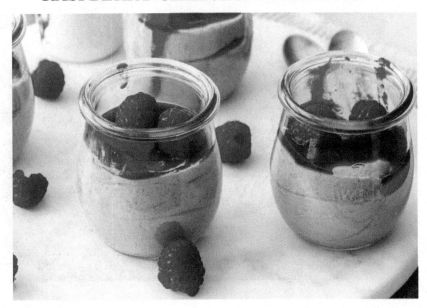

Makes: 4 servings

INGREDIENTS:

☐ 1 cup fresh raspberries

☐ ¼ cup sugar

☐ 8 ounces (225g) cream cheese, softened

☐ ½ cup powdered sugar

☐ 1 teaspoon vanilla extract

☐ 1 cup heavy cream

☐ Fresh raspberries and Mint leaves to garnish

INSTRUCTIONS:

a) In a blender, puree fresh raspberries with sugar until smooth. Strain to remove seeds.

b) Beat softened cream cheese until smooth. Add powdered sugar and vanilla extract, and beat until well combined. Whip heavy cream to stiff peaks in a separate bowl. Gently fold whipped cream into the cream cheese mixture until smooth.

c) Fold raspberry sauce into cheesecake mousse for a swirled effect(reserve a small portion of raspberry sauce for garnish). Spoon mousse into serving glasses; refrigerate for 2 hours to set.

d) Before serving, drizzle the reserved raspberry sauce on top.

e) Garnish with fresh raspberries and mint leaves.

f) Serve chilled and enjoy the creamy mousse.

NUTRITION PER SERVING:

Calories: 400 | Protein: 4g | Fat: 32g | Carbohydrates: 25g | Fiber: 3g | Sodium: 160mg | Potassium: 180mg | Phosphorous: 80mg

MERINGUE KISSES

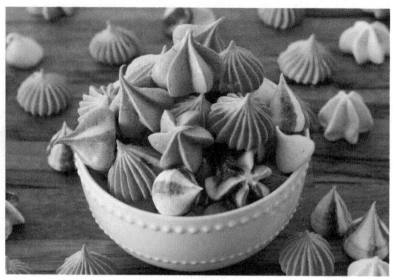

Makes: About 36 kisses

INGREDIENTS:

3 large egg whites, at room temperature

¼ teaspoon cream of tartar

¾ cup granulated sugar

1 teaspoon vanilla extract

¼ teaspoon almond extract (optional)

INSTRUCTIONS:

a)Preheat your oven to 225°F (110°C). Line two baking sheets with parchment paper.

b)In a clean, dry mixing bowl, beat the egg whites with an electric mixer on medium speed until frothy.

c)Add the cream of tartar and continue to beat until soft peaks form.

d)Gradually add the sugar, one tablespoon at a time, while continuing to beat. Once all the sugar is added, increase the speed to high and beat until stiff, glossy peaks form.

e)Add the vanilla extract (and almond extract if using) and gently fold it into the meringue using a spatula.

f)Transfer the meringue mixture to a piping bag fitted with a star tip or any desired tip.

g)Pipe small kisses onto the prepared baking sheets, leaving some space between each.

h)Bake in the preheated oven for 1.5 to 2 hours or until the meringues are dry and crisp.

NUTRITION PER SERVING:

Calories: 20 | Protein: 0.4g | Fat: 0g | Carbohydrates: 4.8g | Fiber: 0g | Phosphorous: 6mg

CRANBERRY TORTE

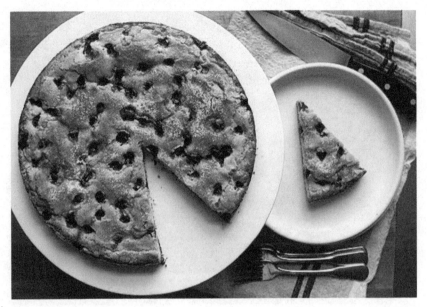

Makes: 8-10 servings

INGREDIENTS:

☐ 2 cups fresh or frozen cranberries

☐ 1 cup granulated sugar

☐ ½ cup unsalted butter, melted

☐ 2 large eggs

☐ 1 teaspoon vanilla extract

☐ 1 cup all-purpose flour

☐ ¼ teaspoon salt

☐ ½ cup chopped walnuts (optional)

INSTRUCTIONS:

a) Preheat the oven to 350°F (175°C). Grease a 9-inch pie dish.

b) In a medium bowl, mix cranberries and sugar; spread evenly in the pie dish.

c) In another bowl, whisk melted butter, eggs, and vanilla extract until well combined.

d) Gradually add flour and salt to the wet mixture, stirring until smooth.

e) If using, fold in chopped walnuts.

f) Pour the batter over the cranberries, spreading it evenly.

g) Bake for 40-45 minutes or until a toothpick comes out clean from the center.

h) Allow the torte to cool before serving.

NUTRITION PER SERVING:

Calories: 250 | Protein: 3g | Fat: 13g | Carbohydrates: 32g | Fiber: 1.5g | Sodium: 70mg | Potassium: 70mg | Phosphorous: 60mg

CHIA SEED PUDDING WITH MANGO

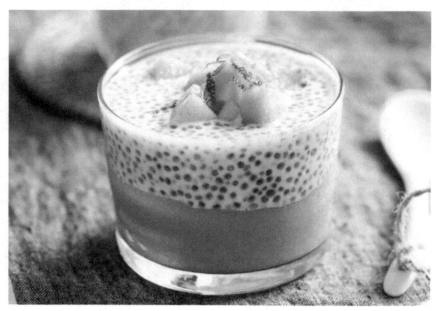

Makes: 3 servings

INGREDIENTS:

☐⅓ cup chia seeds

☐1 ½ cups unsweetened almond milk

☐1 tablespoon honey

☐1 teaspoon vanilla extract

☐1 ripe mango, diced

INSTRUCTIONS:

a)In a bowl, mix chia seeds, almond milk, honey, and vanilla extract. Stir well.

b)Cover and refrigerate for at least 4 hours or overnight.

c)Before serving, stir the chia pudding and top with diced mango.

NUTRITION PER SERVING:

Calories: 180 | Protein: 4g | Fat: 8g | Carbohydrates: 25g | Fiber: 9g | Sodium: 60mg | Potassium: 180mg | Phosphorous: 120mg

VANILLA POACHED PEARS

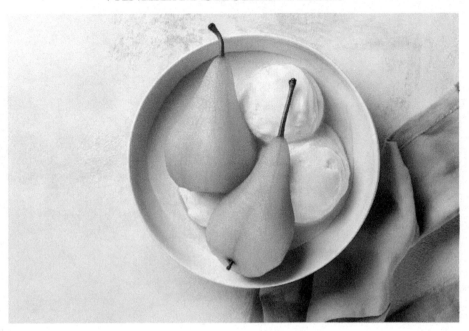

Makes: 4 servings

INGREDIENTS:

☐4 ripe but firm pears, peeled and halved

☐2 cups water

☐½ cup unsweetened pear juice

☐1 vanilla bean, split

☐2 tablespoons honey

☐1 cinnamon stick

INSTRUCTIONS:

a)In a saucepan, combine water, pear juice, vanilla bean, honey, and cinnamon stick. Bring to a simmer.

b)Add the pear halves to the poaching liquid and simmer for 15-20 minutes or until tender.

c)Remove the pears and let them cool. Serve chilled.

NUTRITION PER SERVING:

Calories: 140 | Protein: 1g | Fat: 0.5g | Carbohydrates: 35g | Fiber: 6g | Sodium: 5mg | Potassium: 200mg | Phosphorous: 20mg

FROZEN BANANA BITES

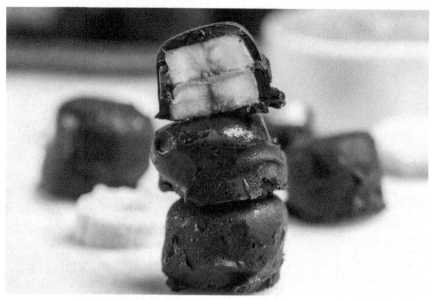

Makes: 2 servings

INGREDIENTS:

☐ 2 ripe bananas, peeled and sliced

☐ ¼ cup unsweetened peanut butter

☐ ¼ cup dark chocolate chips (low-phosphorus)

INSTRUCTIONS:

a) Spread peanut butter on banana slices and sandwich them together.

b) Place banana sandwiches on a parchment-lined tray and freeze for 1-2 hours.

c) Melt dark chocolate chips in a microwave or on the stovetop.

d) Dip frozen banana bites into melted chocolate and return to the freezer until the chocolate hardens.

NUTRITION PER SERVING:

Calories: 180 | Protein: 3g | Fat: 10g | Carbohydrates: 25g | Potassium: 300mg | Phosphorous: 60mg

CONCLUSION

In closing the pages of "Nourish Your Kidneys: The Essential Cookbook for Renal Health," we invite you to savor the fulfillment that comes from embracing a culinary journey intricately woven with wellness. This cookbook, a testament to the dedication in every recipe, extends a heartfelt farewell with the hope that it has not just filled your kitchen with delightful aromas but has ignited a flame of well-being within.

As you embark on the exploration of these delicious and nutritious recipes, remember that each dish carries the essence of a thoughtful approach to managing kidney disease. It's not merely a compilation of culinary instructions; it's a manifesto of care, a guide to improving your diet, and a catalyst for enhancing your overall well-being.

May the flavors linger on your palate, and the nourishment seep into the very fabric of your health. "Nourish Your Kidneys" is not just a cookbook; it's a companion on your path to thriving health and a celebration of the vitality that comes from making mindful and delicious choices.

Here's to the joy of nourishing your kidneys and to the vibrant well-being that follows each delectable bite. Happy cooking, happy nourishing!

RECIPE INDEX

Made in the USA
Las Vegas, NV
09 April 2024